Social Policy in a Changing Society

D0139631

Social Policy in a Changing Society is a critical guide to theories about society, exploring the links between social theory and social policy. It considers a range of interpretations of changes in society, politics and the economy, and assesses their implications for social welfare.

The book is constructed in three parts. The first part considers conventional models, including Keynesian thought, Marxism, liberalism, conservatism, social democracy and socialism. The second part turns to new paradigms, including communitarianism, post-Fordism, globalisation, postmodernity, the risk society, critical theory, Foucauldian thought and patriarchy. In the third part, the authors review debates on social, economic and political change. The approach is mainly theoretical, with material drawn from sociology, political theory, economics and public and social administration.

Social Policy in a Changing Society will be essential reading for those studying social policy and sociology.

Maurice Mullard is Senior Lecturer in Social Policy at the University of Hull. **Paul Spicker** is Senior Lecturer in Political Science and Social Policy at the University of Dundee.

Social Policy in a Changing Society

Maurice Mullard and Paul Spicker

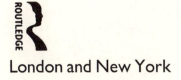

London and New York

First published 1998
by Routledge
11 New Fetter Lane, London EC4P 4EE

Simultaneously published in the USA and Canada
by Routledge
29 West 35th Street, New York, NY 10001

Typeset in Times by BC Typesetting, Bristol
Printed and bound in Great Britain by
Redwood Books, Trowbridge, Wiltshire

British Library Cataloguing in Publication Data
A catalogue record for this book is available from the British Library

Library of Congress Cataloging in Publication Data
Mullard, Maurice, 1946–
    Social policy in a changing society/Maurice Mullard and Paul
  Spicker.
        p.   cm.
    Includes bibliographical references and index.
    1. Social change.   2. Social policy.   I. Spicker, Paul.
  II. Title.

101.M845 1998
    361.2′5–dc21   97-53073
                                                    CIP

ISBN 0–415–16540–7 (hbk)
ISBN 0–415–16541–5 (pbk)

To Alison and Dominique

Contents

Preface

This book has two main aims. The first is to examine the importance of different analyses of society for social policy. There has been an explosion of literature covering new theoretical approaches, but most of it says little about how it relates to social policy. Perhaps as a consequence, new theoretical material – like writing on discourse or oppression – tends to be judged by its moral appeal rather than its intellectual rigour or application to circumstances. The second aim is to bridge the gap between theory and practice. The theory which is currently taught in social policy courses is often abstruse (like the concept of postmodernity) or treads wellworn paths (like the discussion of ideology). The main use of social theory in the study of social policy is to explain the context in which issues are formed and policy is developed. The book examines a range of interpretations of changes in society, politics and the economy, and considers their implications for social welfare.

The basic question the book is addressing is: how do changes in society affect social policy? The approach is theoretical, with material drawn principally from sociology, political theory, economics and public and social administration. Although there are extended discussions of some key topics – such as unemployment, the market, inequality, and citizenship – their main purpose is to help to explain the theories rather than to stand as a treatment of these subjects in their own right. Examples and illustrations, drawn from a range of countries, serve a similar purpose.

The book was written jointly. The initial idea for the book came from Maurice; we agreed a plan together; then Paul dovetailed material written by the two of us into a unified draft. Neither of us would agree with everything in the book, but we hope that the inclusion of strongly expressed, and sometimes opposed, views will make the book livelier and more interesting to read. Any mistakes are, of course, the other one's fault.

Maurice Mullard
Paul Spicker

Chapter I

Introduction

Thinking about society

Theory and practice

Understanding society is mainly done in two ways. One is to begin with observations about society, and then to try to interpret those observations – identifying patterns, trends and relationships for the information which observation makes available. The second main way is to theorise about society, suggesting ideals and then seeing to what extent the social world can be interpreted in those terms. These methods are not really different; they are two sides of the same coin. There is a constant interplay between theory and observation; observations lead to changes in theory, while changes in theory alter what we look at, and how we do it.

Social science

The study of society is sometimes referred to as 'social science'. Science tends, for many people, to conjure up a picture of people in white coats in laboratories who use computers a lot, and social scientists do not really conform to the image. Nor, for that matter, do people who tramp through the Amazon looking for new kinds of beetle, but they are scientists too. Some writers tend to talk about science as if it were founded on only one approach, the generation and testing of hypotheses. But science is based on a range of approaches: much of what happens in the life sciences is based in an ordered interpretation of discovered phenomena, and the basis of biology is taxonomy – the ordered classification of living organisms. Social science, similarly, rests as much on observation, classification and analysis as it does on generating and examining theory. Science is based in reasoned and methodical inquiry, and people who study society use many of the same approaches and techniques as people in the natural sciences. These approaches include observation – the collection of information about the world; the selection, ordering and classification of data; analysis, or the attempt to identify and explain relationships between phenomena; and the construction of theory, which consists of generalisations that can be applied to empirical phenomena.

Some views of science begin with the process of observation. They include induction, which is generalising from observations; objectivism, which searches for the 'real' truth among the facts; and puzzle-solving, a view of science as a search for the answer to problems. Others begin with theory. The most important are instrumentalism, which argues that theories are generated and held for as long as they are useful; and falsificationism, which means that scientists produce theories or 'conjectures' which can be tested, and use them until they are falsified. There is a constant interaction between theory and empirical data, which means that most of these accounts are plausible as a description of how scientists work, but falsificationism, developed by Karl Popper,[1] also explains the process of interaction. It involves forming theories about data, examining data further to see whether the theory still holds, changing the theory as necessary, and testing it again. This is the best expressed and reasoned account of scientific enquiry, and many social scientists apply its criteria.

The central requirement is that a theory has to be capable of falsification, which means that it needs to be put in a form that can be tested and shown to be wrong. A scientific approach sets out to disprove something, not to prove it. Many of the theories in this book, however, are not falsifiable. It is not possible to 'prove' that we are or are not individuals, that private enterprise increases freedom or the capitalist system exploits people, that mutual aid should be thought of as altruistic or that communities are important. These are matters of interpretation; the basis of the interpretation is at root a value-judgment, and depends on normative criteria – the application of moral codes to circumstances. This is a general problem in any attempt to apply social science to social policy. However, the study of social policy cannot avoid moral judgments, and the application of normative criteria is an accepted part of the study of the subject.

The uses of theory

Social policy is much more concerned with practicalities than it is with ideas, and the study of social policy has never been particularly taken with theorising as an exercise. There are good reasons why this should be so. It is not always necessary to understand a problem in order to do something about it and, whether or not we do understand why problems occur, the way into a problem is not always the way out of it. There is a strong pragmatic tradition in social policy, which says basically that one uses what works and drops what does not.

Social theory serves three main purposes. It helps, first, to describe what is happening in society by putting the material into some kind of classification or order. Second, theory makes analysis possible, by identifying the relationships between different factors and explaining what is happening. Third, theory makes it possible to work out principles for action.

The kinds of theory which this book is concerned with tend to be theory on the grand scale, and sometimes these theories seem remote from practical considerations. The discussion depends on a range of concepts, mainly drawn from politics, economics and sociology. We are discussing issues like the nature of a person, of society, social relationships and the influence of economic factors on social behaviour. This kind of concept sets the terms in which other kinds of argument are subsequently framed. As a preface to the discussion of broader social theory, then, it seems important to explain the terms which are used in discourse about society.

Social action

Theories about society have to begin from an understanding of what society is. Some writers have objected to the very idea of society: Oakeshott argues that the idea of 'society' assumes association or set of relationships between people within explaining what the relationships are,[2] a comment which is difficult to sustain after the most minimal reading in sociology. The problem of 'social action' lies in the attempt to explain how people come to act, not as individuals, but as groups, communities or societies.

The individual and the person

Many analyses of society start with the 'individual'. An individual is, more or less, a human being, who can think, make decisions and act on them. Although most people in western society would recognise themselves as 'individuals', the term is very vague. If we mean by it that we have our own thoughts, feelings and actions, it is a half-truth. We are not born, and we do not live, in isolation from other people, and our ideas, feelings and actions reflect the ideas, feelings and actions of other people around us. The idea that we are individuals is not, then, particularly persuasive from a sociological viewpoint.

The value of the idea of the individual is twofold. The first part is political. Individualism argues that every person has to be treated distinctly from others, and that each person's wishes, feelings and thoughts have to be respected. When the idea came to the fore, in the period known as the 'Enlightenment', individualism was a radical doctrine, used to challenge the established world order. The effect of emphasising each person as an individual is to oppose systems that treat people as parts of a greater whole. This was true of feudal society; in the twentieth century, it was true of opposition to fascism. In recent times, the argument has been used by feminists to oppose the subordination of individual women within the household, and by civil rights campaigners wishing to oppose discrimination on the basis of race.

The second part is that, for the purposes of social science, we can analyse some issues by assuming that people are individuals. This is referred to as 'methodological individualism'. Economists describe and predict economic behaviour by assuming that each individual acts independently, and that the actions of individuals can be aggregated to explain the behaviour of the whole. Although most economists would recognise that the assumptions are artificial, the differences in individual behaviour are largely unimportant when the aggregates are considered, and it becomes possible to make statements about the average person – 'homo economicus'. This kind of generalisation can be dangerous, because this average person is not like real people: the average person in economics is not female, never undergoes major changes in his life, and never dies.[3] This can obscure the implications of policy for people who are untypical, and social policy is particularly concerned with the situation of minorities.

In sociology, a 'person' is a different thing from an individual. A person is someone who occupies social roles in relation to other people. Roles are patterns of behaviour, which govern the relationships of people toward each other. Examples might include being a parent, a doctor, a daughter, a teacher, a patient, or a neighbour. These all describe relationships, but beyond that they convey expectations about the ways in which people will behave in a particular context. A role might be seen as a type of 'performance',[4] or as a norm establishing rights and duties towards other people.

The statement that a person occupies roles may seem to say very little in itself; we all occupy roles as part of living in society. The central point is that the roles define the person. To a sociologist, Dahrendorf writes, the person is the sum of his roles.[5] It is from our social relationships that our actions and our existence acquire meaning, both to others and to ourselves. This view of people has been criticised for its failure to take into account other aspects of human knowledge and experience,[6] but it offers nevertheless an interesting insight into the nature of the 'individual'; we are social animals in a sense which is much deeper than that of belonging to a collection of people.

Collective action

A group in society is not simply a number of people. Having common features or characteristics is not enough to make a 'group' in the sociological sense; people with false teeth, or people who eat muesli for breakfast, do not constitute 'groups' (except from the rather specialist point of view of dentists or people who sell breakfast cereal). There are two main types of social group. First, there are people who are linked to each other by a set of social relationships, like a family, a neighbourhood or a workforce. Second, there are people who occupy common positions in society, as defined by their social relationships: women, racial groups or poor people, for example, may be considered to be groups on this basis. A status group consists of people who have a common status – that is, a set of roles, which are associated with common expectations, rights and responsibilities.

Social action by the first kind of group can consist of common action: a family can move house, a neighbourhood can celebrate, a workforce can go on strike. However, people who occupy common social positions do not in general act in common – one of the great myths of radical politics has been that the whole working class would act as one, which even with very considerable organisation is exceedingly unlikely – although the effect of similar social relationships is often to produce similar patterns of behaviour. This is the basis, for example, of women's domestic role and the division of labour in the household – though it should be noted that women in different places have never had quite the same understanding of what the division of labour should be.

Collective action consists partly of common action, but also of mutual actions – actions which members of a group do to each other. As part of social relationships, people undertake duties and responsibilities, which alter the way they behave towards others. The behaviour of a family, or an organisation, generally consists not of everyone acting in the same way, but the outcome of different, interconnected actions in which each person has a role.

Social norms and deviance

Despite the limits to common action, within a society there may be considerable conformity in attitudes and behaviour. Our ideas are not formed in isolation; we are socialised into a range of beliefs, thoughts and patterns of behaviour. The principal mechanism by which this takes place – the unit of 'primary socialisation' – is the family; secondary socialisation takes place through contact with other people, including school and workplace; and tertiary socialisation, more remote than either of the others, is encouraged by the educational curriculum, the mass media or religious instruction.

This means that in any society, people learn how to behave, and absorb views, beliefs from a considerable common fund. People tend to ascribe them to 'common sense', a phrase which puts the situation fairly precisely; it is 'common' because it is held by many others, and drawn from them. These are views which people may not have thought about individually, but which have been learned almost unnoticed from others around them. Berger and Luckmann describe such views as 'inter-subjective'; they are part of a shared set of experience.[7] Edmund Burke referred to this kind of view as 'prejudice' – views where someone's mind is made up before considering the issue – but unlike most modern writers who write about prejudice, he argued that this was a necessary and desirable part of social life. Prejudice, Burke argued, is of ready application in an emergency; it previously engages the mind in a steady course of wisdom and virtue, and does not leave the man hesitating of decisions, sceptical, puzzled and unresolved. Prejudice renders a man's virtue his habit; and not a series of unconnected acts.[8]

The negative side of prejudices is obvious, so it is important to note that it has a positive side as well. We cannot walk around in a state of perpetual moral turmoil, like someone in one of Sartre's novels, having to decide every time we go into a supermarket whether or not we should pay for the shopping or steal it. Parents try to teach children to choose the right things, but most also try to teach them do the right things without thinking.

Social norms are rules which are shared inter-subjectively by many people in a society – not necessarily everyone, but enough to make it a reasonable expectation that people in that society will conform to the rule. Most people do not steal when they shop for food; most people get dressed before going out. More than that, most people do not even think about stealing or going out without getting dressed, because the norm dictates the expectation.

Social norms are important not only for the effect which they have on behaviour, but for their impact when people breach the expectations. The breach of social norms is called 'deviance'; a deviant act is not simply an act which is different, but one which breaks a rule.

Systems and structures

The previous section outlines briefly some of the elements from which sociological analysis is constructed. The next step is to move from these basic building blocks to understanding something about the relationship between them. The structure of a society depends on how these elements relate to each other, and what kinds of pattern they form. Structure can be seen as a metaphor, the imposition of a simplified way of thinking over a complex, shifting mass; it can also be seen as a form of social reality, true both because it reflects the dominant pattern of relationships and because relationships in turn are shaped by it.

Because societies are complex, any simple pattern cannot reflect the whole. Some theories of society, like Marxism or radical feminism, select key characteristics – respectively, class and patriarchy – and argue that these are fundamental in their importance and their impact. Others, such as the 'organic' view of society favoured by some conservatives, focus on the complexity of society in itself as the basis for an argument that society cannot be understood. In sociology, there is also a sceptical approach, called 'phenomenology'. Phenomenology argues for viewing each part of social action as happens, without reading into it interpretations and meanings drawn from other social issues. Each phenomenon needed to be 'bracketed off' from those around it, and examined in its own terms. Phenomenology became important as a means of criticising models of the social order; many of the radicals who espoused it on that basis seemed not to realise that the method was just as destructive of grand theory, like Marxism. Phenomenology is currently out of fashion: the destructive dismissal of wider social relationships is inimical to sociological reasoning, and after one has dismissed preconceptions, it is still important to reconstruct some kind of theoretical insight. (It is still possible to encounter references in sociology to 'deconstruction', which is used in a similar way.)

Modelling

The most commonly used method in the description of social structure is the use of models, or 'ideal types'. A model is a way of describing a set of features in simplified terms, to which reality can then be compared. One of the best-known examples in social policy is the distinction between the 'residual' and 'institutional' models of welfare. In the residual model, the role of welfare is confined to a safety net for people who are unable to manage by other means; in the institutional model, welfare is accepted or institutionalised as a normal part of social life.[9] These are simple, manageable generalisations, and are widely used on that basis.

Modelling can be much more sophisticated than this; the numbers of principles and elements can be multiplied, until the model forms a complex, composite whole. There are, however, problems in the approach. The first, and most obvious, point is that models cannot mirror the real world very precisely. Simple models tend to be vague, and to miss important features. Complex models avoid these problems, but become vulnerable to others. Society is still more complex than the model, and important elements and relationships may be missed. This means that many models tend to describe reality only in part, and there is a tendency to emphasise the features which conform to the model, rather than those which do not. The idea that the private market is motivated by the pursuit of profit, for example, has been so widely accepted that the large areas of private sector activity which are not motivated by profit – such as mutualist insurance, building societies or the voluntary hospitals – are simply ignored.

The central problem with complex models is that the relationships between the parts of the model are assumed to be constant. Because selective benefits are generally associated in Britain with residual welfare, the stigmatisation of recipients and limited resources for welfare, some writers have assumed that these issues are linked. It does not follow that the same relationships have to apply elsewhere. Esping-Andersen's description of 'welfare régimes' describes the main patterns of welfare provision as being 'liberal', 'corporatist' or 'social democratic'.[10] Australia is classified as 'liberal', along with the USA, because some of the features of the Australian system – particularly its emphasis on means-tested benefits – correspond to the *laissez-faire* and residual approach associated with liberalism. Australian writers, however, have responded that the system has extensive coverage[11] and a major impact on the distribution of income,[12] which is inconsistent with the general associations of economic liberalism.

The economic analysis of behaviour

Economics is principally concerned with the analysis of complex interactions, and it has responded to the problems of analysing such interactions in two main ways. One is to select particular elements of the interaction and to work out how that element works, subject to a range of assumptions (or 'parameters'). Each assumption is then varied in turn, to see what effect the assumption has on the basic relationship. From this it is possible to derive certain generalisations about behaviour (for example, that when prices increase, demand falls), which are subject to exception when the conditions do not hold true. Economists who write about policy issues, unfortunately, often tend to forget the assumptions under which the basic analysis was made. An example is the writing of some economists about rent control, who believe that the effect of limiting rent must be to diminish the supply of rented housing.[13] This is only true if other things are equal; the demand for renting is conditional on other factors, including the supply of public housing, the existence of alternative tenures, and the cost of owner-occupation.

The second means is to represent the different elements in a complex situation in mathematical terms, usually as an equation of the form

$$x = \alpha p + \beta q + \gamma r + \delta s \ldots + \text{a constant}$$

This kind of analysis is very useful, but it depends generally on the assumption that p, q, r and s are independent of each other (which may not be true), and crucially on the assumption that the different elements have a cumulative effect. This assumption is potentially misleading, because the elements may have different implications depending on circumstances. It may be difficult, for example, to distinguish the relative impact of unemployment and incapacity benefits in these terms, because in some circumstances they can act as substitutes for each other.

Systems approaches

One of the most important methods available for analysing complex relationships is the systems approach, also called 'systems theory' – though it is a method, not a theory. A system is a way of describing a complex set of interrelated phenomena. Systems are described in terms both of the elements of the system, and of the relationships between them. Each element in turn can be treated as a 'sub-system', in which the key elements and relationships are identified separately. The human body, for example, can be described as a whole, but it can also be discussed in terms of a range of systems – the skeleton, the nervous system, the digestive system and so forth. Society, in the same way, can be said to be a system composed of sub-systems (like family, community and workplace).

Systems approaches are useful as a means of ordering description, and describing relationships. At the same time, they do affect the interpretation of material; they tend to shift attention away from particular issues towards the overall context, and although the relationships are theoretically important, it is much easier to refer to the elements than it is to the relationships. Sociologists have become suspicious of systems approaches, partly because they have learned to be cautious about assuming connections between complex social phenomena – the main message of phenomenology – and partly because the method was much used by functionalist writers, who were believed to be conservative. (The method was also much used by some Marxists, notably Althusser;[14] methods can be associated with certain ways of thinking, but this is not one of them.)

Social structure

The idea that society has a 'structure' is a way of saying that there are certain definable elements in society which have a definable relationship to each other. This proposition is not universally accepted – there are individualists who argue that there is no such thing as society – and among those who accept there is a structure, there are still very great differences in how this structure is seen and interpreted. Some theorists see social relationships primarily in terms of conflict: there are continual tensions, or 'contradictions' (the Marxist term). Others have focused on the nature of social order: the means by which social norms are formed, society is maintained, and social relationships are reproduced for the future. These, of course, are two sides of the same coin, and the division between conflict and order is an artificial one. Marx, the archetypal theorist of conflict, began from the proposition that society was based on the oppression of one class by another – an explanation which requires a developed social order, and the mechanisms by which oppression can be maintained. Talcott Parsons, who occupies an undeserved place in the demonology of modern sociology because of the widespread (and wholly mistaken) belief that he was not interested in conflict, began from the question: why, given all the tensions and problems, does society not fall apart? and constructed a theory of order to help to explain it.

Social division and stratification

The conflicts, tensions and divisions which are evident in society present no problem for individualists, who expect that everyone will pull in different directions; they are problematic for those who want to view society in terms of a system, with structural relationships between the parts. The divisions can be represented in a number of ways. Some divisions run horizontally, so that society is said to be 'stratified', with each layer separated from others above or below them. This is the characteristic pattern of division of social classes; the strongest example, however, is the division of a caste system, in which people are not allowed to move from one layer into another. Some divisions are vertical, running from top to bottom in a society. Linguistic, religious or tribal divisions, of the kind which have riven Belgium or Northern Ireland, can be seen in this way (though it is sometimes argued that such divisions are really economic divisions, and that linguistic or religious differences simply conceal the social reality).

The description of these differences as 'structural' says nothing more than that they fall in an identifiable pattern of social relationships in relation to each other – a view which would still be denied by ardent individualists. Some analyses, however, argue that such patterns are structural only when they relate to key forces in society. The Marxist analysis of society, for example, argues that the structure of society has to be understood in relation to the economic base. Critical social policy is based on a view of society as based in structural inequalities, of which the most important are the divisions of class, race and gender. This emphasis would be justifiable in terms of lack of welfare alone but, for many on the political left, the structure of inequality also relates to the structure of power. Some of the theories that we will consider later are concerned with the way that power fosters or perpetuates social division.

Reading theory: a note

There are some common problems in reading and understanding theories of the kind discussed in this book. First, many of the theories seem remote from the realities of social policy, and they can be difficult to apply in practice. That is one of the main reasons why we felt a book like this might be useful. Second, many of them are vague. Because they are conceived at a very general level, writers are inclined to leave readers to fill the gaps in for themselves. This sometimes means that people read meanings into theoretical works; the trend has been very visible in Marxism, where the considerable sophistication of the readers, by contrast with the lack of subtlety and inconsistencies in the original texts, led to some dazzling interpretations. Many students will have been baffled by their teacher's enthusiasm for some obscure thinker, and assume that they just do not know enough to see what is there. Perhaps the emperor has no clothes.

Third, many of the works on which this kind of book is based are badly written. There are thinkers who can't resist a good phrase, whether or not it makes sense; so, Jean-Jacques Rousseau, often a marvellous writer, began *The Social Contract* with the ringing phrase, 'Man is born free, but is everywhere in chains',[15] which sticks in the memory but has nothing to do with what comes after it. Some writers do not try to make things clear to their reader: Talcott Parsons is reputed to have thought he was such a genius that he ought not to alter anything once he had set it to paper. And some writers, unfortunately, just don't know how to write. Ulrich Beck, whose work on a 'risk society' is terribly fashionable at the moment,[16] *continually* emphasises *key words* in italics (two or three in every paragraph) to show they're important to him, but he does nothing to explain the emphasis – it is left to the reader to invest them with a meaning.

All this calls for some healthy scepticism. Readers should not expect everything to make sense. They should not assume that they don't understand because a greater mind than theirs has spoken. Theory thrives on suggestions and incompletely worked out ideas; if a thought seems unclear, it may just be that it's still only half-baked.

Part I

Old paradigms: how we used to think of society

Chapter 2

Keynesian economics

Keynesian economics was at the root of much that happened in post-war politics. Keynes was an economist, who developed a new paradigm in economic thinking. In a letter to Bernard Shaw, Keynes himself emphasised that his economic ideas represented a revolution in thinking about how economies work.

> I believe myself to be writing a book on economic theory, that will largely revolutionise, not, I suppose, at once but in the course of the next ten years – the way the world thinks about economic problems.[1]

Unlike many theoretical economists, Keynes used economics to construct practical solutions.

> He was . . . essentially an applied economist, a man of action, seeking the best solution of a practical applied economic problem . . . I can remember no occasion on which he tackled a theoretical problem which did not have an immediate practical solution.[2]

His approach to economics was based on narrative and argument, by contrast with the more recent emphasis on mathematical economics, econometrics and model-building. Keynes did not direct his economics at the economic profession since his primary aim was to persuade those outside the profession:

> action required persuasion. And since he wanted action, he wrote not in the esoteric languages of economic jargon or of mathematics for a few colleagues but in the language of those

whose comprehension and support were necessary to the achievement of action – the politicians, the bankers, the civil servants, the financial journalists, the reading public.[3]

The economics of Keynes is of direct relevance to the student of social policy. It questions the received assumption that governments cannot buck the market and argues that policy-making involves political choice. Keynes politicised economic issues which classical economists had tried to depoliticise by arguing that people had to live with the laws of the market.

Keynesian economics provides a framework for intervention in the context of the market economy, because it undermines the previously held view that markets adjust in the long term. Markets might adjust, but not in a way which promotes welfare and well-being. The argument has been made that reducing wages, deregulating labour markets and minimising trade union influence, would create a framework that could generate employment. Even if this was to work, it might not be desirable if a group of workers who are integrated in the labour market find themselves earning low wages in low-skilled jobs in the periphery of the labour market. The Keynesian perspective suggests it probably will not work, and offers in its place a different kind of approach. Generating employment through social consensus, rather than the discipline of the market, could be considered a better and a more socially acceptable alternative.

Keynes and the classical economists

The classical economists argued that the economy was self-regulating. Adam Smith had made the case that the economy was guided by the 'hidden hand' of market forces.[4] The classical model argued that production and consumption in an economy had to balance: in the famous dictum of 'Say's law' that 'supply creates its own demand'. Real unemployment, similarly, was impossible, because the workings of the economy would bring the supply of labour into line with the demand for it. The market guaranteed full employment, defined as employment where everyone who wanted to work was able to do so. That meant, of course, that if people were unemployed, it could only be because they did not want to work.

The classical analysis of the labour market represented it as a balance of supply and demand. If the price of labour increased, the supply of labour would increase, but demand for labour would fall. If the price of labour fell, the supply of labour would fall, and the demand for labour would increase. In the 1920s, Pigou had argued in favour of cuts in wages to resolve the problem of unemployment.[5] Like other classical economists, Pigou argued that unemployment was attributable to high wages and the impact of trade unions on wage stickiness. Pigou pointed out that wage reductions would reduce the cost of labour, which in turn would increase the demand of labour and reduce unemployment. Keynes's response to Pigou was to show that a fall in wages would lead to a fall in overall income thus reducing demand. Reducing demand would lead to a fall in production, which would in turn increase unemployment further.

When Keynes introduced the *General Theory* in 1936, it represented a fundamental challenge to the classical paradigm. Keynes was challenging the assumptions which were 'implicit' to the market model, and argued that whilst market economics presented economic decisions as a series of inevitable outcomes, economic policy actually involved politics and policy choices. He explained in detail why and how the classical economists were wrong. Many of the technical arguments have been a source of rich confusion among economists, and they are too complex to review adequately here. The central thrust of the technical arguments was an explanation of the process by which disequilibrium could arise. Keynes treated different aspects of economic analysis – in particular, employment, interest rates and money – as independent from each other, and questioned whether they were likely to be in balance at all. The classical economists argued that supply and demand would adjust to changes in prices. Keynes argued, by contrast, that if producers found that they still had goods which were unsold, the producers would seek to maintain the price level and so would choose to reduce output which meant reducing the number of people employed. This would lead to further deflation – the loss of real output – because those who would have lost their jobs now had less consumer power. This meant less demand and more goods left unsold, which in turn led to further falls in output.

The second plank of the argument was the imbalance which arose from decisions about savings and investment. In the classical model, savings and investment are equivalent, and the effect of saving now is to create the potential for growth in the future. Keynes sought to show that, in a monetary economy, there was no guarantee that the level of planned savings would be matched by the level of planned investment. People save in relation to their income, while investors are influenced by market expectations and interest rates. If planned savings exceed the level of investment, not all available resources will be fully utilised. In the labour market, the inflexibility of wage structures would ensure that labour markets would not be responsive. There would be unemployment because of the lag in the adjustment between wages and labour supply. In other words, the classical economists believed that saving and prudent housekeeping were the route to growth; Keynes saw them as a fetter on development.

Keynes also argued, crucially, that even where there were processes which would lead back to equilibrium – the 'hidden hand' – they did not have to act straightaway. The classical economists might be right in their belief that output would adjust to prices, but in Keynes' view this would happen in the longer term after a long period of adjustment, deflation and unemployment. Markets would adjust in the long run, but in the long run, as Keynes famously said, we are all dead. This undermined not only the central assumption of equilibrium between supply and demand in the goods market, but also the assumption of equilibrium between savings and investment and the supply and demand for labour. Whilst classical economists assumed that unemployment is voluntary because workers will choose leisure rather than employment at a given wage rate, Keynes argued that unemployment was involuntary because the unemployed had no influence on the wage rate or the demand for labour, and they had no real choice whether to work or not.

Keynesian economic policy

At the core of Keynesian economics was its use of macro-economic analysis – the analysis of the whole economy, rather than just the parts of it. Classical economics was founded on a concept of markets which were made up of the actions of many individuals. Keynes did not ignore individualistic perspectives, but the main thrust of his concern was how they worked in aggregate, for society as a whole. Unemployment was a form of waste, in which people were left doing nothing, and had still to be supported. He wrote,

> It is curious how common sense . . . has been apt to reach a preference for wholly wasteful forms of expenditure rather than for partly wasteful forms . . . For example, unemployment relief financed by loans is more readily accepted than the financing of improvements.[6]

In other words, it would be beneficial to pay people for doing something, rather than to pay them for doing nothing. Full employment was a policy priority, because of the destructive impact of unemployment on the people who experienced it.

> Personal liberty without the full employment of all our national resources is still uncivilised. Less-than-full employment of resources is not wasteful but it also strikes at the heart of community values and the spirit of excellence. Jobs provide people with the basis for the practice of excellence in a very important sphere of their lives. For our society and others, occupations also play a part in creating individual roles and developing personal dignity . . . for it is barbaric to require that certain people in society be denied employment . . . A nation which thrives on the hardships of its members cannot be called civilised.[7]

The Keynesian argument went beyond, though, condemnation of unemployment as it affected unemployed people. Unemployment was an issue for the whole economy. Economic actions had wider repercussions; there was a 'multiplier effect', in which the ripples from each action reached far beyond the immediate scope of the action. The money which was available to one person would be spent with another, who would spend with another, and so forth. The reduction of expenditure in one area would mean that people had less money to spend in another; that meant that reducing public spending was likely to be deflationary (in the sense of reducing output overall). Conversely, increasing public expenditure was reflationary (that is, liable to increase output). Keynes wrote: 'Pyramid building, earthquakes, even wars may serve to increase wealth'.[8] The paradigmatic example of this was gold mining. Gold mines were an obvious waste of time and effort – mining employed lots of people digging for useless metal – but the economic repercussions could fuel an expansion of the economy as a whole.

Armed with this analysis, Keynes made a modest proposal to produce something nearly as good as a gold mine.

> If the Treasury were to fill old bottles with banknotes, bury them at suitable depths in disused coal-mines which are then filled up to the surface with town rubbish, and leave it to private enterprise on well tried principles of *laissez-faire* to dig the notes up again . . . there need be no more unemployment, and, with the help of the repercussions, the real income of the community, and its capital wealth also, would become a good deal greater than it actually is. It would, indeed, be more sensible to build houses and the like; but if there are political and practical difficulties in the way of this, the above would be better than nothing.[9]

Keynes's prescription was startling – but it worked. Keynesian policies became strongly associated with programmes of public works, adopted in the 1930s with great success in Roosevelt's America and Hitler's Germany. And this led to great confidence, in the post-war period, that governments knew how to deal with unemployment, that they could support the economy constructively, and that they could help to promote economic growth and development. This was the dominant wisdom for thirty years, until the oil crisis of the 1970s led to the reemergence of market liberalism.

Keynesian economics – not the economics of Keynes himself, but the school of thought developed in the post-war period around his approach – was strongly linked with the idea of demand management. The role of government was seen as a means of moderating the instability of the economy. When the economy was growing, in a 'boom', there was a risk that over-production would lead to retrenchment and reductions in planned investment, and this in turn would send the economy downwards. Once the economy was in a 'slump', there was no necessary reason why it should turn up. Demand management was intended to moderate the booms, to achieve steady, stable growth, and to encourage growth during a slump. In political terms, however, damping down a boom is difficult to justify: the characteristic pattern of the British economy in the 1950s was described as 'stop–go', basically the pattern of a semi-managed economy which was being perennially interfered with for political advantage.

The welfare state as constructed after 1945 rested on the assumption that governments would adopt a Keynesian approach to macro-economic policy: namely, that there would be a commitment by governments to maintain 'full employment'. This commitment to full employment made possible the welfare state designed by Beveridge and implemented by the 1945 Labour Government. The principle of insurance could only be made to work if there were high levels of employment and the unemployed were going to experience unemployment as a short-term problem. High levels of unemployment and long-term unemployment would therefore always undermine the major pillars of public finances. Those in employment had to generate the finances necessary to fund health, education, pensions and other major areas of social policy. If on the other hand unemployment levels started to rise, government would lose finance because of loss of taxes but also would have to pay high levels of social security to the unemployed. Furthermore, this was also likely to have major effects on pension contributions.

The importance of Keynesianism for welfare is difficult to underestimate. Keynes was called, in his day, 'the man who saved capitalism'; he was also the man who provided the central justification for the expansion of welfare services as a key to industrial achievement and performance. Keynesian macro-economic policy was essential to the welfare state. It was assumed that commitments to full employment would generate economic growth, high levels of consumption and higher tax yields to finance welfare expenditures. The welfare state could be used as an instrument of macro-economic policy. Increased expenditure on infrastructure, including roads, communications, social housing and hospitals, would improve areas of social policy but would also generate employment and contracts for private-sector companies. Employment in the public sector would also contribute to the wider economy. And social protection for the poor would act as a regulator for the economy, increasing public expenditure in times of deflation, and reducing it again during recovery. A discussion of the post-war welfare state which does not refer to Keynes is like Hamlet without the king; there's still a lot going on, but the issues wouldn't make a lot of sense.

The problem of inflation

Despite its considerable success, Keynesianism did not offer the answer to everything. One remarkable example was the construction of Brasilia, which began in 1957. In order to get a new capital built, the Brazilian government printed money to pay for it. This was a classic Keynesian programme of public works, which in principle should have helped to develop the Brazilian economy. It did so. It also, however, led to two thumping great problems: a massive rate of inflation, and a huge debt which Brazil (like many other developing countries) was in no position to repay. Brazil's economic problems were a major reason for the military coup of 1963. For many of the critics of Keynesianism, inflation was its Achilles heel, and ultimately it was a concern with inflation which led to its abandonment.

Inflation is concerned with the value of money rather than the level of economic activity. Inflation is a process of steadily rising prices which results in a reduction of the purchasing power of a sum of money. The opposite of inflation is *disinflation* (not, as some people assume, deflation). There is, however, a link between deflation and disinflation. The level of money in the economy is an indicator of the demand for goods, and demand stimulates production. When the amount of money is reduced – for example, by reductions in public expenditure – demand falls, and so does the level of economic activity. Conversely, increasing expenditure may generate inflation, but it may also increase demand and so help to reflate the economy. Inflation and disinflation are concerned with the value of money; reflation and deflation were concerned with the level of activity in the real world, and unemployment reflects what is happening in the real world rather than the money markets. Keynesianism never said that inflation led to growth. Inflation is, at its most simple, a problem of 'too much money chasing too few goods'; it may happen not only because there is too much money, but also because there are too few goods. There is no necessary connection, then, between inflation and employment; inflation can happen because the economy is under-performing, as well as when it is cooking. A healthy economy can have low unemployment and low inflation. But the belief that this was not possible undermined the will of governments to remove unemployment, in the belief that this could only be achieved at the expense of financial stability.

Wage inflation and unemployment

The Phillips curve was an attempt to show that full employment could only be bought at the expense of inflation. Although it was widely taken to be a Keynesian argument, it seemed to establish a fundamental flaw in the Keynesian approach. Phillips argued that there was a direct connection between the level of unemployment and the rate of wage changes.[10] When unemployment was low, wages would rise fast due to the competition for labour. When unemployment was high, wages would fall – though they would fall less rapidly, because of worker wage-resistance. The evidence for the Phillips curve has never been strong: Ormerod notes that there is no stable relationship between unemployment and inflation, and reviews evidence that 'it is not in fact possible to find a regression linking inflation and unemployment over any length of time after the First World War which is at all satisfactory.'[11] Nevertheless, the argument that there was such a relationship has proved profoundly influential.

Friedman argued that the Phillips trade-off was based on the assumption that workers only bargained around nominal wages.[12] People are sometimes misled by the apparent value of wage increases. This is referred to as 'money illusion'. Friedman contended that workers might suffer from money illusion only in the short term. In the long term therefore they would bargain for real wages. Because agents bargained on real wages, bargains were likely to be struck around the expected rate of inflation and the expected real wage. The higher the expected rate of inflation, the higher the level of nominal wage inflation consistent with a given expected real wage and level of employment. The trade-off between unemployment and inflation was not stable. Because of the presence of inflation, and workers trying to compensate for future inflation, it was more accurate to argue for an augmented Phillips curve which showed an unstable and increasing trade-off between the unemployment rate and inflation.

The central assumption in this analysis is that inflation is fuelled by increases in wages. Some economists have seen trades unions as a thermometer reflecting inflation; others have represented them as having a 'furnace effect' rather than a 'thermometer effect', where pressure for increased wages is seen as the cause rather than the consequence of inflation. Keynes was concerned that full employment would lead to pressure on wages, and he took the view that this was a political rather than an economic problem:

> Of course I do not want to see money-wages soaring upwards . . .
> It is one of the chief tasks ahead of our statesmanship to find a

way to prevent this. But we must solve it in our domestic way, feeling that we are free men, free to be wise or foolish.[13]

Keynes had argued that his concern was with economic problems and that unemployment was an economic issue. Whether full employment was compatible with holding down wage inflation represented a different problem:

> I do not doubt that a serious problem will arise as to how wages are to be restrained when we have a combination of collective bargaining and full employment. But I am not sure how much light the kind of analytic method you apply can throw on this essentially political problem.[14]

Keynesians have seen the process of inflation reflecting a series of relationships between firms which can mark up prices, the impact of trades unions on wages, inflation and government. These can be described in terms of three processes:

1 the wage–wage spiral, which reflects a context of competing wage claims within different sectors of the economy, the impact of decentralised bargaining and wage drift;
2 the wage–price spiral, where the rate in wage rises squeezes out the profit margins which in turn leads to firms marking up their prices; and
3 the price–wage spiral, which occurs through shock increases in prices such as the oil price increases in 1973 and 1974 which resulted in workers attempting to increase their wages to protect their take-home pay.

Incomes policy became central to a Keynesian economic strategy. Within the context of an incomes policy all three agents make certain commitments to achieve an enduring social contract. Growth in the economy is redistributed into investment, wages and the social wage.

> An incomes policy is not just a device for limiting the wage gains of organised workers. Rather, it represents a means of determining the annual, non-inflationary rise in all the different types of incomes that accrue to households. . . . Moreover, in a democratic society an incomes policy cannot be imposed. It

must gain acceptance among the different economic interest groups as the fairest and most equitable basis for distributing the fruits of technological progress.[15]

It seems to follow from this argument that unemployment might have to be raised in order to hold down inflation, and if governments chose a policy of low inflation then the policy cost of low inflation was high unemployment. Equally, if government adopted policies to reduce unemployment then they had to live with rising inflation. In this sense economists were able to establish a trade-off between unemployment and inflation, in contrast to the classical view that unemployment was a problem of market rigidities and inflation a problem of government. The idea of a 'non-accelerating inflation rate of unemployment', or NAIRU, became popular. There is no evidence to support the idea that there is such a rate: rather, Ormerod suggests, any constant level of inflation can be maintained with any constant level of unemployment.[16]

A primary emphasis on wages belies the complexity of the issues. Inflation does not simply reflect the cost of labour, and the relationships described by the Phillips curve have not been consistently reproduced. Inflation is a general problem of rising prices, and rising prices can be fuelled by many factors: they include profits, rents, the money supply, interest rates, rates of exchange, the availability of capital, production (because scarcity leads to higher prices), and the costs of primary goods. The increase in oil prices in the 1970s was not the result of rising wages in developing countries, and nor was the inflation which followed it.

Keynesianism in the global economy

Goran Therborn has argued that the central reason why some countries were more able than others to cope with the recession and unemployment of the 1980s were the differences in institutional arrangements in these countries to manage economic policy.[17] The author points out that in those countries which had established and mature institutionalised agreements, unemployment was less severe than in those countries which had relied on market forces.

Underlying the variations there seem to be two common important patterns, which are certainly inter-related. One is the remarkable national unity around a set of concrete policy priorities . . . Secondly, largely because of this consensus, there appear to be strong expectations by all important actors in the successful countries that there will be a fairly long-term continuity in basic government policy orientation.[18]

However, the vulnerability of the Keynesian-managed economy to changes in the international markets points to a much more fundamental challenge to Keynesianism than the concern with inflation might suggest. Keynes's analysis was based on a closed economy – an economy in which there was an identifiable set of repercussions for each action. The wider the scope of the economy, the less true this may be. Increasing demand in one economy could be met by increasing numbers of imports, rather than increased production. The multiplier would not be contained within a region, and government action could not be guaranteed to stimulate activity only within the boundaries of a nation-state. This has encouraged some economists to focus on stimulation of selected industries – 'supply-side' economics rather than demand-led. This meant, in turn, that policies for economic development could not necessarily rely on the benefits of welfare expenditure.

These problems are felt acutely in the developed economies, where global links are of considerable importance. The International Monetary Fund and World Bank were initially set up with Keynesian objectives – indeed, Keynes himself was the principal designer of the IMF. The IMF was intended 'to contribute . . . to the promotion and maintenance of high levels of employment and real income and to the development of the productive resources of its members', while Keynes described the World Bank as existing 'to develop the resources and productive capacity of the world with special attention to the less developed countries, (and) to raise the standard of life and conditions of labour everywhere.'[19]

The problems of Keynesianism in the developed world have meant, however, that for developing countries which are attempting to join the world economy, Keynesianism has not been an option. The IMF and World Bank have promoted the need for 'structural adjustment'. In general, structural adjustment refers to the need of developing economies to adjust to the conditions of the global economy; in practice, it is associated with a range of policies, including the reduction of fiscal deficits and public expenditure, especially expenditure on welfare. The IMF's stabilisation programs, Watkins comments, 'are almost always designed to reduce demand, notably by cutting government expenditure, controlling money supply, and raising interest rates, stringent targets being set in all of these areas.'[20]

In a traditional Keynesian analysis, the effect of this within local economies would be to deflate the economy, forcing industry into a slump. Unfortunately, this seems to be pretty much what is happening.

The politics of Keynesianism

The economics of Keynes was important for social policy at both an intellectual and a practical level. At an intellectual level the Keynesian argument went beyond a technical argument with classical economics. Keynesians sought to offer a revolution in thinking about government and economy and therefore aimed to break with the classical paradigm that a *laissez-faire* economy was the only solution for the well-being of a society. Keynes showed that the market economy left to itself could not be trusted to generate sufficient investment and employment. While agreeing that markets would tend to clear in the long run, the long run was always going to be achieved at high social costs. Since life was too short, it was morally right for government to intervene and, therefore, reduce the sufferings of mass unemployment. Keynes also showed, through the concept of the marginal propensity to consume, that governments could redistribute income to lower income groups in a way that contributed to economic prosperity as well as to social justice.

The political arguments of the Keynesians were no less influential than the economic ones. Keynes used his position as an economist to oppose the dominant political views of his time. The classical economists presented the market in terms of immutable laws. This implied that governments had little or no autonomy in the conduct of economic policy, except to create a framework where markets could flourish. This was strongly associated with market liberalism, in its acceptance of the economic status quo. Keynes was dismissive of these arguments, which in his view were based on ignorance about economic processes. He wrote: 'Practical men, who believe themselves to be quite exempt from any intellectual influences, are usually the slaves of some defunct economist.'[21] By contrast, Keynes argued that the major concern of government was to discover ways of improving welfare and general prosperity. 'The outstanding faults of the economic society in which we live are its failure to provide for full employment and its arbitrary and inequitable distribution of income.'[22] Societies are continuously faced with choices in responding to economic issues, so that although the economy appears as a series of exogenous factors, it is always within the sphere of political choice as to which policies are selected or prioritised. Economic policy alternatives always represent political choices.

An essential element in Keynesian economics is the assumption that individuals are capable of carrying out wider social contracts, and the recognition of interdependence rather than instrumental contracts based on self-interest. Keynesian economics can therefore be seen as being founded on assumptions of mutuality, of the ability and willingness of individuals to relegate their self-interest to the wider social interest. A form of continuous contract can be constructed between the state and other key agencies in society. Implicit in the economics of Keynes are the concepts of civic virtue, social justice and democracy. In one sense, therefore, Keynes was committed to the concept of the Greek polis and the view that progress depends on dialogue and reason. According to this approach reason is made possible through communication, through trust, listening and being persuaded by the argument of others.

Keynesian economics integrates ideas of civic virtue and political democracy. This would suggest that societies can have trades unions, social security and full employment with low inflation, if unions are willing to recognise the equation of entitlements and obligations. This means a willingness to recognise that those entitlements to social security benefits, trades union rights and stable employment also require a series of obligations, including the obligation to moderate wage demands, to trade-off wage demands for other social benefits such as social security and pensions. It is the recognition of entitlements and obligations which provide the opportunity for a civilised economy.

The welfare consensus

Daniel Bell wrote about the 'end of ideology' in the 1950s.[23] It seemed that the all-embracing theories of the world – communism and fascism – had failed, and that *laissez-faire* capitalism was a thing of the past. Governments managed their economies, and knew what to do with them. The Keynesian orthodoxy was at the root of that. In retrospect, the consensus is more difficult to identify. There were ideological divisions, and many of the ideological arguments reviewed in this book were developed in the very period when consensus was presumed to reign. But there was also substantial agreement in the formal politics of many western countries about the purpose of government intervention, which was for the public benefit; the capacity of governments to bring about socially desired effects; the economic and civil rights of citizens; and the development of social protection – a guarantee in case of socially recognised need. Many political disagreements focus on the method by which these principles could be applied. The depth of agreement is most visible in the reaction to political systems which did not accept these principles – like South Africa under apartheid, which made government an instrument of racial oppression – or to those which were believed to have subordinated the public benefit to other kinds of principle, such as religious fundamentalism or political ideology.

Keynesian economics needs to be located in the context of a form of politics by consent, of government seeking to secure an economic policy through consensus building. This legitimised the importance of functional groups in the making of economic policy. Because the commitment to full employment requires economic agents to make certain concessions, the process of government becomes a series of bargains between groups and the government. Governments therefore became increasingly dependent on vested interests. Often, in the view of critics of this kind of government, this was at the cost of those individuals whose interests were not represented by the strategic groups involved in the policy process: Keynesian economics was dominated by groups involved in production. Keynesianism came to stand for the 'corporatism' which has characterised many European governments: the co-operation and negotiation of factions under the umbrella of the state.

In political terms, corporatism is a form of interest-group representation, which mediates the activity of different factions through the brokerage of the state. For some, it is a pluralist model, based in co-operation and consensus; others see it as a means of exercising power through the medium of non-state agencies. Schmitter describes corporatism in terms of 'a limited number of singular, compulsory, noncompetitive, hierarchically ordered and functionally differentiated categories, recognised and licensed (if not created) by the state'.[24]

It is easy to dismiss the idea of corporatism as a political 'consensus', because continuing conflicts in society are all too evident. But political consensus does not mean that conflicts are not present; it means that they are not formally recognised, which is a different issue entirely. The consensus refers to acceptance of the rules of the game, how the game will be played, and to some extent what it will be played for. Bachrach and Baratz, in *Power and Poverty*, criticised just this effect; within formal political processes, certain issues were kept off the political agenda, contrary views were suppressed or translated into a more acceptable structure, and dissidents were co-opted into the political process.[25]

The view that the consensus has broken down reflects the resurgence of ideology, and in particular the emergence of the 'radical right'. In a range of countries – including for example Britain, the USA, Sweden and New Zealand – political movements have arisen which dispute the principles of the consensus on the role of government, the effectiveness of Keynesian economics and the legitimacy of welfare. (These views are considered in more detail in Chapter 4.)

In that light, it is interesting to note a phenomenon which characterises the role of welfare in a number of countries: the issue of 'convergence', the spontaneous harmonisation and conformity of different social systems. For example, most OECD (Organization for Economic Cooperation and Development) countries have moved to social protection through insurance in the event of old age and sickness, and complete coverage of the financial costs of medical care in hospitals. There are several reasons for this: they reflect common social problems, including ageing populations and the issues of dealing with unemployment in formal economies; common approaches, reflecting cultural diffusion; a degree of technological determinism, for example where the received pattern of western medicine shapes the delivery of medical care; and direct imitation of the policies of other states. The phenomenon of convergence points to the continuing power of received wisdom and orthodoxy within industrial countries. The breakdown of the consensus does not mean that there is no more orthodoxy; but that orthodoxy is no longer Keynesian.

Chapter 3

Marxism

Marxism in theory

For many years, Marxism dominated academic discussion of particular issues on the left, and although fewer commentators would now refer to themselves as 'Marxist', the influence of Marxism is still evident in the vocabulary which is used to discuss social issues. Sociology as a discipline was also profoundly influenced by Marx; the main opposition to Marxist analysis was Weber, and Weber drew on and modified a Marxist vocabulary – terms like class, capitalism and power – as a means of arguing against Marx's position and conclusions. The effect was, however, that much of the debate was framed, and sustained, in the language of Marx.

There is a basic problem in outlining and explaining Marxism. Marxism was not just a social theory, and not just a political doctrine, but a system of belief. For those who followed it, it explained everything important in life, including family, sexuality, art, culture, politics and religion; it predicted the future; and it provided a sense of worth and a social life. As a social theory, Marxism was never very satisfactory. Despite his dogmatic claims to be 'scientific', Marx's reasoning was often obscure; he expressed himself in inconsistent and sometimes contradictory terms, and his predictions were inaccurate. In the hands of intellectual Marxists, Marxism became much more sophisticated, and a force to be reckoned with: it was used, not as a theory, but as a flexible set of tools and arguments to provide an analysis of society, and it is on that basis that it needs to be considered here.

The materialist base of society

Marx's thought was based in a materialist view of society and history. The central view is that the nature of economic production determined the pattern of relationships in a society. The structure of economic production – the 'forces of production' – shaped the relations of production, or the role which people had in the economy. The forces and relations of production together produced a substructure of society, which was then reflected in everything else, including politics, culture and intellectual activity. 'As in material, so in intellectual production', Marx wrote;[1] he was explicit that the way we think is produced by society, not the other way round.

> The mode of production of material life conditions the social, political and intellectual life process in general. It is not the consciousness of men that determines their being, but, on the contrary, their social being that determines their consciousness.[2]

The economic determinism which this implied was the source of much criticism. Many later Marxists, and people seeking to revise Marxism, chose (like Gramsci and Lukacs) to emphasise the interaction between economic factors and ideas, or (like Baudrillard and Habermas) to argue that the process of change could move in the other direction, from culture to the structure of production.

The key to understanding the relations of production was simple enough: they were the relations of oppressor to oppressed. In every developed society, production took place because some people exercised power over others. Slavery gave way to the feudal system, and the feudal system gave way to bourgeois production, or capitalism, but the fundamental character of all of them was the same – the exploitation of one group by another. This is why Marx wrote that 'the history of all hitherto existing society is the history of class struggle'.[3] Classes were groups of people defined by their relationship to the means of production.

Marx referred to his argument as 'historical materialism'. The historical element came because the engine of social change was conflict between the social classes. As the mode of production changed, so did productive relations; each system gave birth to another, which in time would destroy it. The feudal system was destroyed, Marx argued, by the emerging bourgeoisie, a new class concerned with commerce and industry. The bourgeoisie, in turn, would be destroyed by the new working class, the proletariat, which would revolt and take over the state. The victory of the proletariat would mark the end of the process, by establishing a new and different kind of society based on equality and flexible production rather than oppression.

In this conclusion, there were two basic inconsistencies. First, if all of history is based on oppression, and each dominant class is replaced through an inexorable logic by another dominant class, it should follow that the bourgeoisie would be replaced by a new kind of oppressor, and not by the proletariat at all. (Karl Popper argued that if there was a revolution, on Marx's own premises the revolution would itself lead to the dominance of a new class.[4]) Second, if the development of society was determined by its mode of production rather than by political system, a revolution which seized the political system could not address the fundamental issues. Marxism was, explicitly, a system for revolutionaries; it coupled exhortations to revolution with the argument that the outcome was inevitable, and arguments to say that things would never change through politics with demands to do precisely that. Resolving these contradictions is not very important for our purposes, but it may help to explain something of the approach which Marxism took.

This also meant, however, that Marxists had a problem when the predicted outcomes failed to materialise, and even those Marxists who did not feel they had to accept the precise terms of Marx's analysis have often fallen prey to the temptation to treat the predictions as carved in stone. Marx said that the capitalist system was incapable of improvement, and that people must become miserable under it. Marxists have consistently emphasised the failures of the industrial system, and dismissed its successes. Marx said that the system would inevitably collapse, and for the last 150 years Marxists have been arguing that the system was in a crisis and that economic collapse was imminent. Marx said that after capitalism there would be the revolution, and since we have not had the revolution it follows that what we have now must still be capitalism. These are quasi-religious beliefs, and they have proved to be no more susceptible to counter-argument than beliefs in astrology or spiritualism.

Capitalism

The central issue in Marxist analysis was a view of modern society as 'capitalist'. Capitalism was distinguished by the dominance of capital, a system where certain people owned and controlled the means of production – though Marx commented that capitalists were simply 'capital personified', which suggests that the means of production controlled them. Capitalism was motivated through self-interest and the pursuit of profit by private individuals.

This is not actually a very good description of the industrial process in the present day. In the first place, profits are not necessarily made by private individuals; firms are owned by other firms. The largest bloc of shareholders on the stock market in the UK are pension funds, which are managed on behalf of pensioners who have no say in how they are used. The people who own the means of production, then, are not necessarily those who control it. Second, industry and commerce are not exclusively private, as they once were. Anthony Crosland, in *The Future of Socialism*,[5] emphasised the importance of the role of the state in the control of the economy and the ownership of industry. This role may seem to have diminished since Crosland's book was written (the precise extent of state intervention is debatable), but the central argument still holds good. What has happened is that the '*laissez-faire*' which was the basis of nineteenth-century capitalism has long ceased to apply (if it ever really did). States intervene actively in modern economies, as planners and managers, producers, consumers and distributors of resources; the ability of industrial firms and financial organisations to act for themselves is conditioned by government policy, and in some countries government is involved intimately in decisions on management and investment. Third, because ownership and control have been divorced, the industrial process has come to depend on managers – a trend which was visible even in Marx's time, though he dismissed it. Managers' interests often differ from those of the shareholders. Most managers are interested in personal incentives, job security, and status, which may lead them to pursue long-term growth or the advancement of personal careers rather than the profits of the organisation.

The exploitation of labour

Marxism described the capitalist process in terms of a division of labour in which some people had to sell their labour power to others in order to produce goods, and were exploited for the surplus value of their labour. Value was produced by the labourer, but the capitalist made a profit by buying labour and selling goods at a higher price. This was made possible by paying the labourer less than his true value – the exploitation of the labourer.

The labour theory of value is based in some important misconceptions – for example, that labour, rather than the value of an object in use, determines value, or that only the labourer is adding anything of value. At the simplest level, it fails as a description of the productive process: most people who are involved in economic activity are not actually producing anything. They are administering, servicing, organising, or assisting the few people who are producing something. This is a system of production in which production is socialised rather than individual; it makes an analysis in terms of the exploitation of individual labour power fairly meaningless.

No less fundamentally, this misses much of the point about social injustice. Kymlicka comments:

> What about those who are forced not to sell their labour? Married women have been legally precluded from taking wage employment in many countries. Hence they are not exploited . . . Or consider the unemployed, who are legally able to accept wage employment, but can find none. They too are not exploited . . . Something has gone wrong here. Exploitation theory was supposed to provide a radical critique of capitalism. Yet, in its standard form, it neglects many of those who are worst off under capitalism, and actually precludes the action needed to help them (e.g. welfare support for children, the unemployed, and the infirm).[6]

Marx sought to deal with the last point by justifying some collective redistribution of resources from a common pool,[7] but there is an underlying contradiction in this: if people have a basic personal right to what they produce themselves, it is difficult to justify taking it away from them. That is precisely the argument made by market liberals.

The accumulation of capital

Marxists saw the central trends in capitalism as being the accumulation and concentration of capital. In order for capital to be accumulated, the economic conditions have to be created in which goods can be produced and traded. The first step is the development of a formal market economy, which is one of the key issues in studies of the Third World; subsequently capitalists demand the conditions in which production, and so profits, can best be made. Marxists have emphasised the creation of conditions of accumulation as one of the key issues in the operation of the capitalist economy. Saunders points to the role of the state in

> Sustenance of private production and capital accumulation . . . by aiding the reorganisation and restructuring of production in space (e.g. planning and urban renewal) . . . through the provision of investment in 'human capital' (e.g. education in general and technical college education in particular) . . . through 'demand orchestration' (e.g. local authority public works contracts).[8]

The accumulation of capital depends on the establishment and growth of markets, and so on supply and demand. Neo-Marxists have emphasised the importance in this of 'commodification',[9] turning activities into the kind of thing which can be bought and sold in the market. House construction, for example, is not commodified in much of the Third World, where people construct their own squatter shacks and then progressively improve them; but it is commodified in most developed countries, where people buy land and materials and commission builders to construct houses for them. The development of mass industrialised housing, notably tower blocks, took this trend to an extreme; industrialised building methods centred control in particular firms which were equipped to deal with them.

The welfare state is often seen as decommodifying things, or taking goods and services out of the market. Offe argues that decommodification is necessary to compensate for the problems which arise from production, to reproduce society, and to legitimise the system: 'a supportive framework of non-commodified institutions is necessary for an economic system that utilises labour power as if it were a commodity.'[10]

At the same time, it is possible to argue that much of what happens in the welfare state favours the conditions of accumulation, implying commodification rather than decommodification. Wherever people are given cash benefits rather than goods, they have to engage in market transactions.

The concentration of capital

Marx argued that capital would become concentrated progressively in fewer and fewer hands. He outlined the process by which a revolution would come about as involving first, the accumulation of capital; second, its concentration and 'centralisation', as some capitalists became richer and richer at the expense of everyone else;[11] and finally progressive immiseration, as the ranks of the proletariat swelled and capitalism denied them basic resources, leaving them no choice but revolution.

Marx condemned the tendency to accumulation as being inextricably bound up with human misery.

> within the capitalist system, all the methods for raising the social productivity of labour . . . are transformed into means of domination and exploitation; they mutilate the worker into a fragment of a human being, they degrade him . . . they make work a torture . . . It therefore follows that to the degree in which capital accumulates, the worker's condition must deteriorate, whatever his payment may be.[12]

It should be fairly obvious that this is not what has happened. The industrial economies have created considerable material benefits as well as considerable social problems, and over two centuries the position of the poorest has unquestionably improved. This is not just a matter of historical interest; it remains of fundamental importance in the development of Third World economies, where Marxist analyses still carry a great deal of weight. In the process of economic development, poor people are progressively integrated into the economic system. Although the benefits are sometimes unclear, and there can be casualties in the process, this is the main route through which the living standards of people in developing countries can be improved.

The general trend as economies develop has not been towards concentration: the relationship is described by the Kuznets U-curve, which describes inequality as increasing and then diminishing as economies develop.

> At the early stages of development, both physical and human capital are scarce and unequally distributed. Their owners command high returns on both (scarcity premium). As both types of

capital accumulate and become less concentrated, the rate of return on physical capital tends to decline, while wage differentials between skilled and unskilled labour narrow. Income distribution gets more equal.[13]

The idea that income distribution has become more equal in modern societies will give some readers pause, because in a few societies (and particularly in Britain) there has been an evident increase in inequality in recent years. The problem here is twofold. The first concerns the basis for comparison – the picture looks different over ten years than it does over a century. The second is that the kind of inequality which Marxists are interested in is not necessarily the same as those who are interested in income inequality. Marxism is mainly interested in the division between those at the top and the rest. Here, the figures are much less persuasive. The kinds of inequality which have been increasing are mainly those which divide the bottom third or so from the working population, to the point where writers have been talking about a division of 'two-thirds–one-third' or perhaps '30–30–40' (30 per cent at the top, 30 per cent vulnerable in the middle, and 40 per cent at the bottom). These are very rough descriptions, but they are much better accounts of what has been happening than the idea that we are divided between the bourgeoisie at the top and the rest.

Class

Although the idea of 'class' is used to mean a range of different things, including status groups and people in different economic positions, Marxism has a much more specific understanding of the idea of class. A class is defined in terms of its relationship to the means of production. The most important classes were the bourgeoisie, or capitalist, class, and the proletariat, who were the industrial workers. Marx wrote that society was becoming divided into these two main camps, but he did not think they were the only classes. Other classes in his analysis included the peasantry, who were left over from the former feudal system, and the *petit bourgeoisie* (or small traders). Marx did not think these classes would last; people would be driven into one or another of the main classes. This, like most of his predictions, was not what happened; there are survivals of old arrangements, including peasants and the gentry, minor classes like the *petit bourgeoisie* have survived, new kinds of class have emerged (notably public sector workers), and some people have been displaced through structural changes in the economy (the so-called 'new poor'). There is a case to argue that the bourgeoisie themselves – the people who own and control the factories they work in – are a hangover from an older system, rather than the model for the current society.

For Marxists, the divisions of class were the most important in society, and the only ones that really mattered. The inequalities suffered by women, for example, were largely explicable in terms of the inequalities of capitalism and class. Engels explained the position in terms of class – women's labour in the family was a commodity, in the same way as men's labour was. Engels wrote: 'the real content of the proletarian demand for equality is the demand for the abolition of classes. Any demand for equality which goes beyond that of necessity passes into absurdity.'[14]

Many people have, of course, argued that equality between the classes is nothing like enough: Tawney, for example, was concerned to provide equality in the basic conditions of life,[15] which on the face of the matter seems a much more radical demand. Marxist feminists were generally content to accept this analysis.[16] Later generations of feminists have been less happy to subordinate their position. Heidi Hartmann comments: 'The "marriage" of Marxism and feminism has been like the marriage of husband and wife depicted in English common law: Marxism and feminism are one, and that one is Marxism.'[17]

In recent years, revisionist writers have written about a range of 'new social movements' – concerned with issues like race, gender and disability – which have offered different critical perspectives on current society from the concern with class traditionally identified by Marxism.[18] There is nothing new about these movements; in many cases the arguments have been around longer than Marxism. The main difference is that Marxists have stopped ignoring them.

The Marxist analysis of class was profoundly influential. It shaped the terms in which inequality was analysed, and focused attention on the position of workers as the most basic issue in society. Because of Marxism's political influence, this also meant that the central concern of social policy was to represent and protect the position of the working class. This was particularly visible in continental Europe, where the term 'social' often stands for industrial relations, and trades unions came to occupy an institutional position in the organisation of welfare. The idea of 'social partnership' in France developed welfare provision formally as an area in which employers and workers had a direct interest. For people working in social policy, this approach was both invaluable and infuriating: invaluable because it was fundamental to an understanding of the development of much social provision, infuriating because there was no visible place in it for the poorest and most disadvantaged people. Marx dismissed the poorest people in society, the 'lumpenproletariat', as the 'social scum'; the organised labour movement often had no time for them. The distinction between the working class and the poor has always been important, but Marxism did not really consider it.

The ruling class

The idea of class was more than a means of describing the stratification of society; it was also a description of the structure of power. The 'ruling class' are those who own and control the means of production. This does not mean that they rule by sitting down together to make decisions; the Marxian concept of class unifies people according to their shared interests, and they rule in the sense that they establish the conditions in which government operates. 'The executive of the modern State', Marx wrote, 'is but a committee for managing the common affairs of the whole bourgeoisie'.[19]

Marxists have taken differing views of the relationship of the state to the ruling class. Miliband argues that the state is an instrument of class oppression.[20] This happens in part because the industrial system constrains what it is possible to do in government, but also because people who are responsible for government share the values and priorities of the ruling class. Poulantzas, against this, argued that the state is much more complex: it reflects the conflict of different classes, and of factions within classes. This means that there are likely to be inconsistencies, or contradictions, in state action.

> The State organises and reproduces class hegemony by establishing a variable field of compromises between the dominant and dominated classes; quite frequently, this will even involve the imposition of certain short-term material sacrifices on the dominant classes . . . But . . . all measures taken by the capitalist State, even those imposed by the popular masses, are in the last

analysis inserted in a pro-capitalist strategy or are compatible with the expanded reproduction of capital.[21]

Capitalism and welfare

Marxists usually see the provision of services as the outcome of a conflict between capital and labour. The welfare state is mainly understood as a series of concessions won by the organised labour movement. However, the effect of the dominance of the capitalist class means that such measures are moderated to ensure they are broadly compatible with the aims of capitalists and, in particular, that they do not conflict with the accumulation of capital.

Neo-Marxist writing has tended to emphasise the role of welfare as a means of promoting capital accumulation. O'Connor writes that the welfare system acts to 'expand demand and domestic markets'.[22] Habermas emphasises the role of the state in creating conditions for the 'realisation' of capital, for example:

> through improvement of the material infrastructure (transportation, education, health, recreation, housing construction, etc.); . . . through heightening the productivity of human labour (general system of education, vocational schools, programs for training and reeducation, etc.).[23]

The role of the state is described, in 'regulation theory', as the regulation of economic and social conditions in order to promote the accumulation of capital.

Welfare also has the main function of legitimation. This means that a major purpose of welfare is to make the operation of the capitalist system acceptable, which can happen either through changing the way people think and behave (legitimation through the educational process) or by offering concessions to mollify them. However, the attempt to maintain welfare services is beyond the financial capacity of states. This implies a contradiction between the functions of accumulation and legitimation, most clearly expressed in Habermas's discussion of 'legitimation crisis'. Offe writes, famously, that 'while capitalism cannot coexist with, neither can it exist without, the welfare state'.[24]

There is a range of objections to this approach. The first is that there has to be some mechanism by which this all develops. The basic approach is functionalist; it depends on the attribution of a purpose to existing elements of the social structure. A functionalist analysis calls either for some kind of structure or internal logic which pushes capitalist states in a particular direction, or the conscious use of power to make systems conform. Although neo-Marxist writers have generally opted for the latter explanation, conventional Marxism is more likely to see the emergence of welfare systems as the result of conflict than of systematic necessity.

The second problem lies in the view that welfare is a burden on the economy. This premise is much used by critics on the political right as well as on the left, and it is highly disputable. Spending on welfare does not conflict with economic growth – the Keynesian analysis suggests the opposite – and, although more developed economies tend to have more developed welfare systems, there is no clear association between expenditure on welfare and economic success or failure.[25]

The third problem lies in the idea of 'legitimation'. Why, if capitalists hold all the power, should they bother with public acceptance? Why should welfare go beyond what is necessary to make labour productive? Some Marxists have argued that provision for old people or mentally handicapped people is cursory: Spitzer suggests that such people are treated as 'social junk', because they are unimportant for the productive process.[26] But this is not what really happens; services to old people are central to what happens in welfare states, to the point where Walker writes (with some hyperbole) that 'the welfare state is chiefly a welfare state for elderly people'. Legitimation seems to be a way of dismissing whatever welfare states can provide that is worthwhile. In a previous book, Paul Spicker argued:

> There comes a point at which 'legitimisation', if taken far enough, cannot be regarded as merely instrumental. If legitimacy is gained through acting in people's interests, a state which devotes a high proportion of its resources to the welfare of its citizens is more legitimate than one which does not.[27]

Marxism and social policy

In the context of social policy there are two main Marxist approaches. The first is founded in the structural analysis of *Das Kapital*. Marx tried to outline a series of crisis tendencies which, he argued, would undermine the capitalist economy and bring forward a different economy. Capitalism carried the seeds of its destruction. Marxists who used *Das Kapital* as a starting point tended therefore to see government intervention in terms of responses to the needs of capitalism. Capitalism needed skilled workers and therefore the state intervened to provide an educated and and healthy workforce. To maintain legitimacy the state provided transfer payments for the unemployed and the elderly. Infrastructure expenditure on hospitals, roads and housing could be described as contributing to the accumulation process.

The second approach, by contrast, is rooted in Marx's political writings. Marx attempted to explain the dynamics of class analysis, for example mapping out class forces during the French Revolution. The logic of class suggested that the welfare state was a product of class relations. Interventions which widened the scope of social policy represented victories for the working class, while retreats from social provision represented defeats. The welfare state represented the vortex of class analysis at a specific point.

In response to the retrenchment of the 1980s and 1990s, the logics of capital and class provided competing responses. Marxists who favoured the logic of capital argued that the retrenchment confirmed their analysis. Capitalism was characterised by inherent crisis, and the attempt by governments to create processes of accumulation and legitimacy had created new internal crises. Marxists argued that Keynesian solutions would not deal with the long-term crisis of capitalism. The crisis of welfare and Keynesian economics since the 1970s confirmed that capitalism was displaying problems of decreasing profits and problems of accumulation. The problems of unemployment and recession in the 1980s showed that capitalism could not afford a welfare state. This crisis would force a new phase of socialist thinking and transformation.

By contrast, Marxists who emphasised the importance of class relations explained the crises of the 1980s as confirming the ebbing of working-class influence. In the 1980s working-class movements were on the ebb. Cuts in social provision showed the inability of the working class to defend all the gains that had been made in the post-war years. (The trends were not all in the same direction, however; there was also, during this period, a general trend to the universalisation of health care.)[28] The 1980s confirmed the flow of the ruling class. This was aided by the policies of the New Right whose priorities were to restrain working-class resistance through changing the landscape on trade union reforms. The decline of parties of the left also confirmed the inability of social democratic parties to protect working-class interests.

Marxism: an overview

There is so much wrong with the Marxist analysis of society that it can be difficult to see why it should have exercised such an influence. Part of the reason is, certainly, political: the dominance of Marxism in the Soviet Union and China meant that it seemed to many to represent the only alternative to 'capitalism'. The argument was politically convenient to advocates of the free market, who have often stigmatised any argument in favour of collective action as communist or quasi-Marxist. Part rests in the appeal of an over-arching theory of everything, for those who like an ordered view of the world.

Two elements, though, exercised a particular attraction. One was the claim of Marxism to address issues of social injustice; the other was its claim to represent socialism, and with that to argue for collective action. Both of these claims were bogus. The Marxist treatment of social injustice was inadequate; there was no developed theory of justice, nor even of equality. Dependent poverty was substantially ignored; issues of gender and race were treated as a minor aspect of social class; disadvantaged groups, like people with physical disabilities or elderly people, were ignored or dismissed. Marxism was sufficiently flexible to be adapted to address these issues, but the focus of Marxist thought was always elsewhere, on the 'central' conflict between workers and employers. The second issue, relating to collective action, was diminished and confined by concentration on the industrial sphere. Marxism often claimed as its own a range of different approaches which had other intellectual origins – notably syndicalism, which stood for workers' control. Many of the most interesting forms of radical collective action grew from other initiatives: co-operatives grew from guild socialism and Owenism, community development (in different ways) from the work of anarchists and American liberals, and participative models of politics from liberalism and democratic thought. The diversity in thought and approach which can be found in contemporary critical writing reflects this wide range of sources and influences.

Chapter 4

Liberal individualism

Liberalism and the individual

The starting position of liberalism is that we are all individuals. There is no such thing as a society. What there is just individual men and women, each of whom has their own feelings, thoughts and patterns of behaviour. The individual exists as a reality, exists separately from community and is neither a product nor a part of community. Individuals should be recognised in their own right as knowledgeable and able to make decisions that do not depend on others.

Individualism grew as a radical doctrine. The medieval view of the world put a great emphasis on social order. Everything in the universe had a place and a role. Society was organised so as to put the great above the petty, and each person received what was appropriate to his or her station. (The hierarchical view which this represents has not completely disappeared. Reactions to monarchy – which is, of course, a vestige of feudal society – are still governed by similar sentiments.) The individualism of the Enlightenment was highly subversive. It argued against this ordered, petrified view of the world by arguing for the individual. People had to be judged by their worth, not by their birth. People should have the opportunity to learn things, to rise above their station. Careers should be open to people according to talent and merit. One of the great ironies of individualism is that, despite its radical beginnings, it became over time a means of justifying the status quo – of accepting a society supposedly based on individual action.

In contemporary society, most of us have heard the individualist argument so often that it has lost any power it once had to surprise. However, as a description of society individualism is just not true.

People are not individuals in this sense; we are born into families and communities. We do not have free thoughts, feelings and patterns of behaviour; we are socialised into generally accepted patterns of behaviour, and the way in which we express ourselves and relate to other people is conditioned by our social circumstances. As a moral statement, it has more to commend it. It argues that we should treat each person as worthy of respect; that each person has rights.

This is the starting point for Nozick's book, *Anarchy State and Utopia*. 'Individuals have rights, and there are things no person or group can do to them (without violating their rights).'[1] Nozick believes that there is a natural right to liberty – that is, a right which is not dependent on other people, or on the society of which the individual is part. Action which infringes individual free-dom is prima facie illegitimate. The rights of the individual include rights to life and to liberty – which are generally understood in a negative sense, to mean that other people cannot legitimately inter-fere. In the USA, where libertarianism has been most influential, it seems to be associated with a view of society based on John Wayne films and the myth of the frontier, where people could go and live as individuals without reference to a 'society'. This kind of myth has also spread into green politics through the work of Thoreau; the rural idyll of *Walden* argues that people can be self-sufficient, independent, free spirits.[2]

It is easy to be dismissive of individualism, because much of this kind of argument is, for all its moral claims, simply immoral – a selfish, smug, hedonistic and self-righteous defence of privilege. This is unfortunate, because individualism still has some important points to make. The strength of liberalism rests in the argument that if each person is to be valued and respected, people need to have rights as individuals. The effect of treating people as a mass is that individuals within that mass can be sacrificed for the greater good. Intervention cannot be justified simply because some people gain at the expense of others:

> The moral side constraints upon what we may do, I claim, reflect the fact of our separate existences. They reflect the fact that no moral balancing act can take place among us; there is no moral outweighing of one of our lives by others so as to lead to a greater overall social good.[3]

Social norms are often repressive; the strongest arguments against arranged marriages or female circumcision have been individualist ones. In order to protect everyone, it is important to offer protection for each person.

Two premises have been central to the defence of the individual. The first is the argument that individuals know what is best for themselves. The individual will always be more sensitive to personal needs and to the likelihood that these needs change. The individual is basically rational: the individual has natural competence and technical competence. Natural competence denotes the ability to maximise individual well-being. Natural competence means the ability to be strategic in making choices, since alternatives carry costs, so that natural competence must be the ability to maximise personal well-being at the least possible cost. By contrast, giving the power to bureaucracy or professionals, to define what is needed or to prioritise the needs of society, is likely to lead to less flexibility. It also implies a more homogeneous approach to a situation when individuals need to be treated differently.

Since individuals know best, no one else has the right to announce on behalf of the individual what real need is, nor to put order on preferences or to moralise on behalf of the individual. The role of government should be to provide the context, based on rules which protect the right of self-interest. Government does not encourage a selfish morality by legitimising self-interest, but rather a process which ensures the freedom of the individual against the more arbitrary morality of others.

The second principle is the assertion of the fundamental equality of individuals. This may surprise those who associate liberalism with the New Right's opposition to equality. The argument that men have rights by their nature claims an initial degree of equality – a sense in which people cannot be legitimately disadvantaged.[4] Rae comments that market liberals are not so much anti-egalitarian as narrowly egalitarian.[5] Liberalism advocates the conduct of government through a process of law which ensures equality of treatment of all individuals.

> The great aim of the struggle for liberty has been equality before the law. This equality under the rules which the state enforces may be supplanted by a similar equality of the rules that men voluntarily obey in their relations with one another.[6]

Individual liberty can only be guaranteed if government conducts itself in the context of rules, including a written constitution that ensures the separation of powers within government, and which ensures that majorities do not vote in such a way to erode or put into question individual rights. According to liberals, policy should be guided through a series of rules and principles which are publicised so that the individual is made aware of the conduct of government.

Individualism offers a valuable critical perspective on the way in which society operates. We should not assume that because people on the whole are better off, or because certain groups benefit, that each and every person within that group has benefited. This has been most visible in liberal feminism, which has complained of the invisibility of women within the 'black box' of the family.[7] By examining the position of each member of the family separately, individualists can be aware of the sources of disadvantage and inconsistencies in position which affect some people and not others.

It should also be noted that individualism can have important practical implications. Sheila Shaver, considering the issue of abortion, notes that European countries which nominally have more generous systems of welfare provision and favourable provision for women than the USA may also have more restrictive policies relating to abortion.[8] Abortion is a complex moral issue, in which a series of conflicting norms come into play: they include the rights of the mother, the rights of the father, the rights or interests of the foetus, the position of professionals who conduct the abortion, the interests of society and the imposition of other moral codes, particularly religious ones. The reason why the USA has a more liberal code on abortion is that the individualist ethos represents the issue primarily in terms of the rights of the mother; by contrast, European societies limit the scope for purely individual action, because society and other people are held to have an interest.

Liberalism and equality

The principle of fundamental equality was identified in the previous section. Liberals generally accept that people are entitled to equal treatment, which means not identical treatment but rather treatment without disadvantage, bias or prejudice. Beyond this, liberal thought has also been strongly associated with equal opportunity, and the idea of 'the career open to the talents'. The way to achieve the best use of labour in society is to make sure that people are allowed to become what they are capable of becoming. Equal opportunity ensures that all offices and careers are open to all individuals, that each individual has equal access. The dimension of equal opportunity is related to the principles of efficiency and also natural liberty. A distribution is efficient if no one can be made better off without making someone else worse off; inefficiency implies that people are worse off than they need to be. If the distribution of income acts as a barrier to entry for certain individuals so that these individuals, because of lack of income, cannot explore fully their abilities, then resources are not being allocated efficiently.

Equal opportunity is a complex concept, however. If it means only that people are not prevented from rising, then it is the same thing as equal treatment. Rae distinguishes between equality of opportunity which is prospect-regarding and means-regarding. It is prospect-regarding if people are able to participate in a contest which anyone could win. It is means-regarding if people have the means to gain the end.[9] Liberals have tended to accept the argument for means-regarding equality of opportunity at least in relation to educational opportunity, which is the basis for further opportunities in society.

Inequalities in wealth and income are more problematic. The presence of income inequality can mean that the level of income determines which individuals are more able to utilise their potential. Lack of income acts as a barrier to entry into higher education, and is associated with children from lower income groups leaving school at an early age. If human resources are not deployed effectively because of income, then some liberals would argue that government must address the question of income to improve efficiency. Income inequality is also of concern to liberals for a second reason. Inequality of income is likely to deny natural liberty to some individuals so that some individuals will be less able than others to pursue what they see as desirable and good. Income concentration is likely to lead to the monopoly of vested interests, whose levels of income and property have the potential to influence government and therefore harm the rights of the individual. Conversely, income inequality denies some individuals the right to self-interest. Liberals should, therefore, be concerned with the question of the rights to property and the rights of the individual. Hayek seems to assume that there is no tension between concentrations of property ownership and the rights of the individual. Indeed, Hayek argues against any attempt by government to discriminate in taxation policy. Yet property can also be utilised as a resource by some against the rights of others.

Individualism and property rights

The rights of the individual are often understood to extend to property. It is assumed that property rights reside in the individual, and freedom creates a presumption of non-intervention in relation to individual property. This is a curious assumption. Chopping the end off someone's garden to build a sewer is not at all the same kind of thing as chopping off someone's leg, and it seems very strange to argue that the same principle governs both. Property rights have developed through convention, tradition and legal process; the individual ownership of property is a relatively recent historical development (in Roman law, property was held by families), and there have often been restrictions on trading certain types of property.

Interference with someone's property or goods is treated as equivalent to an interference with their freedom. Some liberals would argue that the rights of the individual are invariably linked to the rights of property. Hayek for example argues that only when the rights to property were established did the feudal monarchies stop treating others as 'subjects' to be used in the service of the monarch and the rights of property and individual rights emerged. Once it is recognised that individuals have a right to their property enshrined in law, others are compelled to observe rights to property.

> An important aspect of this freedom – the freedom on the part of different individuals to pursue distinct aims, guided by their differing knowledge and skills – was made possible not only by the separate control of various means of production but also by another practice, the recognition of approved methods of transferring this control . . . The prerequisite for this existence of such property, freedom and order from the time of the Greeks to the present is the same law in the sense of abstract rules enabling the individual to ascertain at any time who is entitled to dispose over any particular thing.[10]

The right to property and the protection of property is central in guaranteeing the freedom of the individual. Attempts by governments to use their powers to redistribute property therefore must be seen as a form of coercion. Nozick sees redistribution as theft, and taxation as a form of slavery; no state is entitled to remove resources from one person in order to benefit another. (Nozick is, however, prepared to accept redistribution as a form of compensation for past wrongs.[11]) Hayek argues that governments do not have the right to introduce progressive taxation since this form of taxation seeks to discriminate because of income. (Kukathas attributes to Hayek the principle that taxation should be governed by rules of proportionality, so that each individual pays the same rate of taxation irrespective of income.[12] This implies, however, a concern with the distributive implications of policy which Hayek elsewhere dismisses as inappropriate.[13])

The liberty which is being defended here is a very specific kind of liberty. In the first place, it is highly negative; people are held to be 'free' when they are not subject to coercion, not when they are able to do things autonomously. People who are poor are not necessarily subject to coercion, but they are not free, if by that we mean they are able to do things or to make choices. Second, there are good reasons for saying that people's freedom must not be infringed, for example in securing their persons against assault; but in cases where individual property comes into conflict with other concerns, for example in building communal facilities like a road, it is not evident that individual property should be sacrosanct. Third, the argument which identifies freedom with property rights also gives property rights a position of central importance. The value of freedom, Taylor argues, is not as a principle in itself, but in what it allows us to do. Freedom of assembly, freedom of religion or freedom of speech matter more than the freedom to drive at speed; unnecessary traffic controls are a nuisance, but restrictions on worship are a matter of principle.[14] Property rights are important, but are they more important than freedom from want, the right to life, access to health care or education?

The arguments relating to property are, then, only half true. Hayek is probably right to say that property has to be respected, because some kind of property is basic to personal security. But this is not an absolute value; it is one value to be set against others. The main effect of the concentration on property rights has been to turn individualism from a critical and moral perspective into a defence of the status quo.

The role of the state

Nozick argues that individual freedom limits the role of the state: the minimal state is the most extensive state that can be justified. Any state more extensive violates people's rights.[15] The state, the argument continues, is necessary to protect the freedom of the individual from the depredations of others. It has, therefore, basic functions of maintaining order, providing defence, and perhaps to some degree as an arbiter in disputes between individuals. This is the limit to which the state may act: if it extends its influence further, the freedom of the individual is infringed.

Liberals in favour of a minimal state – ultra-minimalists – argue for a constitutional form of government, where the spaces and limits of government are set within a framework of law, and an independent judiciary supervises the rights of the individual and the process of government within that framework of law. The Constitution should establish the rights of the individual in such a way that changes in government will not lead to changes in the rights of the individual. This means that the Constitution should state clearly what the rights of the individual should be. It seeks to expand privatised lives where individuals seek to resolve problems through families, networks, employment and neighbourhood. Individuals are therefore asked to retreat from the public sphere because 'politics' is unpredictable, unstable and unjust.

Other modern liberals have tended to see more of a role for the state. The liberalism of Hayek, Friedman and Brittan does not take for granted that the individual exists in nature but rather that individualism has to be created and protected.[16] According to this argument the individual is not perceived as having some natural existence: the individual needs to be created. It becomes the duty of governments to promote the climate of liberalism.

Liberalism and the market

Liberalism is strongly associated with *laissez-faire* in the economic sphere. *Laissez-faire* means to leave people to get on with it, and that is pretty much what liberal economists believe is best. In establishing the new political economy, the advocates of classical market economics wanted to promote the theme of the natural rights of the individual. Seeking to explain the changes in agriculture during the 1760s, Adam Smith argued that it was not government direction that had been promoting the new technology but rather the process of autonomous individual self-interest. This self-interest was basic to social improvement: 'It is not from the benevolence of the butcher, the brewer, or the baker that we expect our dinner, but from their regard to their own interest.'[17] The state, the monarchy, and feudal society had all acted as constraints on the freedom of the individual, and were prime targets of classical liberal reformers.

In the traditions of market liberalism, markets are both desirable and inescapable. They are desirable because they are responsive to the decisions of individuals; at times the advocates of the market seem to take as given the argument that individuals left to themselves would always choose to live within the context of the marketplace. They are inescapable because whenever people make unconnected decisions, a market will emerge – that is what a market is.

Markets are seen by liberals as self-regulating. Smith wrote of the 'hidden hand' by which the economy would be brought into balance. The market model is constructed according to three general assumptions of the nature of the individual and the relationship between the individual and the wider social context. First, the individual is a rational agent continuously making choices based on rational information. The concept of the rational individual suggests the individual knows best which projects to pursue and also is aware of the costs and benefits involved in making certain decisions. Individuals are continuously making choices. These involve opportunity costs – decisions to forgo some things in order to get others. Because decisions are also related to the state of knowledge which is available, it is likely that with new or additional information the individual might change the order of needs and preferences. Market liberals do not suggest that the individual is socially atomised, but that the individual is located within a specific social and historical context. However, the rational individual is capable of continuously questioning and renegotiating the priorities and preference as set by others.

The second assumption is that the right of individuals to pursue self-interest remains the best way to increase the prosperity and welfare of the individual and of the community. The primary concern is always the right of the individual to be able to make choices free from direction by a central authority. Needs and preferences are best met through markets by individual consumers and suppliers making 'decentralised' decisions in contrast to direction coming from a centralist authority. The market represents the process of the invisible hand, invisible in that there is no overall direction on intervention by one authority to attempt to define what should be produced, how a product is produced and for whom.

Third, the individual is sovereign in the market place, which means that there is freedom of choice and opportunities for individuals to realise their self-interest. This also depends on the view that the market provides a context where people are likely to be treated as equal individuals. Because the market involves many buyers and sellers without barriers to entry, the spirit of competition ensures that individuals who feel discriminated against have the freedom of choice to move to new markets. The potential for discrimination between individual consumers is consequently minimised. It is more likely that discrimination and the perpetuation of vested interests will be maintained in a context of monopoly.

Unemployment

For market liberals, the analysis of the labour market is like the analysis of any other market. Labour is a commodity, bought and sold by rational agents in the market. In an article in the *Financial Times*, Samuel Brittan, the economics editor, drew a comparison between labour and bananas as two similar commodities:

> If the price of bananas is kept too high in relation to the price required to balance supply and demand there will be a surplus of bananas. If the price of bananas is below the market clearing price there will be a shortage. The same applies to labour. If the price – i.e. the wage – is too high there will be a surplus of workers, i.e. unemployment. If it is kept too low there will be a shortage of workers . . . Workers do sell their services just as banana producers sell bananas.[18]

Acting as rational agents, workers will adjust their wages in relation to the level of demand for their level of services. The rate of unemployment represents 'excess' labour supply at a certain wage level. The consumers of labour – the employers – have the right to choose in the goods market because there is competition between suppliers. Where price is the determining factor, the rational consumer will choose the product that offers the highest level of welfare at the lowest price. Furthermore, since the national economy is likely to be an open economy, this means that the consumer can choose between goods produced anywhere in the world. In the context of the open economy, the cost of the goods produced in Britain has to reflect international competition which in turn means that British workers, when setting their wages levels, are also faced by international competition.

The central thesis in market economics suggests that in the climate of competition it is the consumers in the goods market who are choosing which goods to buy, and so who determine the price. The level of unemployment represents the failure of the labour market to clear at prices determined in the goods market and that therefore wages in the labour market have to adjust before labour markets clear at full employment. It is consumer sovereignty in the goods markets which determines prices. A high level of unemployment would indicate that the price of labour is too high and that wage levels would need to be adjusted downwards if labour markets are to clear. If the concept of rational agents is correct and prices are flexible, the question arises as to why there is a lag between unemployment and wages. Why do wages continue to rise irrespective of the level of unemployment? Why do the unemployed not seem to represent a threat to those at work? For some sectors of the economy it seems as if the unemployed might as well be in Newcastle, Australia as in Newcastle, England. They simply do not influence wage demands. The long-term unemployed, those who have been registering as unemployed for eighteen months or more, tend to have low skills, and are not geographically mobile. They are less able to move to parts of the country where there is a high demand for labour.

Market liberals and Keynesian economics

For Keynesians, these arguments miss the point. Keynesians argue that unemployment arises because there is no reason why it should not arise; the economy is not self-regulating. The debate between Keynesians and market liberals continues to reflect the tensions between those who continue to see themselves as disciples of

Keynes, arguing for government intervention, the need to generate civic virtue and a civilised economy, and those who argue that the market represents the only solution to the challenges of the globalised economy.

The market liberal critique of what is seen as the Keynesian era is twofold: there is the argument that first, Keynesian perceptions of government and politics are dangerously naive, and second, that economic policy founded on political choices fails to deliver on economic performance. Whilst Keynesians would argue that the public forum is essential for creating a civilised economy as against the dominance of self-interest, market liberals would argue that such forums actually produce the new barons of corporatism who decide behind closed doors who should get what, when, and how. Market liberals have argued that such decisions are likely to be more arbitrary and unjust than the marketplace and that it was always better therefore to leave decisions to the market and individual self-interest since these are always more likely to be just than those produced under Keynesian corporatism.

In the economic sphere, Keynesianism is seen as the source of a range of problems, including inflation, inefficiencies and unemployment. Within a market liberal framework, unemployment is explained as being a problem of rigidities in the market, the outcome of government regulation and intervention, the impact of trades unions and the levels of social security benefits. To gain employment people have to obey the rules of the market, which means that when the market results in low pay then low pay has to be accepted as the outcome. Contracts are between individuals – the firm is treated as an individual equal to the individual employee. Trades unions distort the process of wage bargaining, because they can be in a monopoly position. Government regulation of contracts similarly distorts the market: employees should not look to government to regulate the hours they work because employees enter into voluntary contracts.

Public choice

The theory of 'public choice' is an attempt to apply economic methods, including methodological individualism, to the analysis of politics. Public choice theory starts from the assumption that all individuals are utility maximisers and therefore seek to maximise their self-interest. Similar to the market for goods and services, in politics there is also a market which is based on identifying those who supply political goods and those who demand political goods. On the supply side are included politicians, public sector professionals, civil servants, governments and political parties, while on the demand side the consumers of political goods include voters, households and sectional interest groups. Those on the supply side are as much 'utility' maximisers as those who seek to maximise their well-being on the demand side. Each is pursuing self-interest. Politicians want to remain or want to become the incumbent government, and voters are seeking increasing public goods provided someone else finances their demands.

The founder of public choice theory was Downs, who built on Joseph Schumpeter's view of democracy. Schumpeter had argued that democracy consisted of a struggle between parties for people's votes, and that such political responsiveness as could be found happened because politicians needed the votes to stay in power.[19] In *The Economic Theory of Democracy* Downs argued that political parties acted as entrepreneurs promising to provide public goods at little cost in terms of taxes to the electors.[20] Downs suggested that voters chose the political party that promised the most goods at the lowest possible price. The implication of Downs' thesis was that governments were likely to under-spend their budgets because voters were likely to put a lower value on public goods. In the market for goods and services, there was a direct relationship between the price and the product. Public goods were one step removed in that consumers could not really identify what they were getting for their money. Brittan argued, in contrast to Downs, that governments would over-spend their budgets because there was a tendency for political parties to 'outbid' each other in making promises to electors during elections.[21] The tendency for politicians to outbid each other meant that the tendency was that governments would continuously increase their budgets while at the same time being reluctant to increase taxes to fund the new additional expenditures.

Public choice theorists including Niskanen, Buchanan and Tullock criticised the Downs model during the 1960s by arguing that the relationship between voters and parties was distorted by other factors which were outside the political system.[22] Niskanen introduced the concept of the budget-maximising bureaucracy. It was in the self-interest of civil servants to expand their departmental budgets, and so they made it their business to persuade the minister responsible for the department to ask for increased expenditure from the Treasury. Civil servants and public sector professionals are in a monopoly position because of their access to information. They are an estate of the realm founded on knowledge – a 'knowledge estate'. In a complex society, ministers have to rely on the advice of their civil servants and the professionals.

Public choice theory also seeks to deal with the impact of sectional interests on public provision. Welfare states encourage the expansion of pressure groups around major areas of expenditure. Pressure groups involved in the poverty business, defence contracts, or agriculture subsidies sustain 'the tyranny of the status quo' through a process of policy inertia and exclusion of others, a process which imposes both internal and external constraints on government and the individual citizen. Public sector trade unions can bargain on wages and conditions of employment directly with government. Because this happens outside the rigours of the labour market, wages become highly politicised, and trade union members can use the strategies of both voice and exit from major public services. Beer argues that the impact of pressure groups leads to a series of scrambles around benefits and pay, eventually resulting in political paralysis and a crisis of governance.[23] Pressure groups try to ensure that maximum publicity is given to their service if government announces cuts or containment in their budgets. They display 'bleeding stumps'. This includes the sudden closure of a hospital by hospital authorities as a means of attracting attention and generating a crisis for the government. School closures, the cancellation of a defence contract and laying off employees are means by which sectional interests seek to advertise their plight, whether the cutbacks are real or imagined.

Those who work in the public sector also make choices through rational self-interest – and in that, they are no different than those who worked for private companies. Public sector employees were also willing to strike to increase their wages and conditions and were willing to utilise their monopoly position as providers of education or health care to get governments to listen. In health care, it is the medical profession which influences the distribution of resources between different health priorities in investing in technologies to deal with cancer screening, heart disease, the care of the elderly. In education, the professionals decide issues of teaching and resources.

Public choice theory questions the view that those who work in the public sector do so because of a commitment to a public service ethic, or that politicians become politicians because they want to serve the public. Those involved in both the demand for services and those who supply public services are doing so out of their self-interest. Politicians like being politicians; they like being the incumbent government. Civil servants and public sector professionals are a knowledge estate and politicians depend on this knowledge for policy analysis and policy advice. The bureaucracy and professionals are able to shape the priorities of public policy working with politicians and leaders of interest groups within the iron triangle that excludes the citizen. This has led, over time, to an increasing emphasis on personal incentives in welfare services, an approach which is very different from an ethic of public service. Julian Le Grand has expressed an important concern about this approach. In an article titled 'Knights, knaves or pawns?' he suggests that treating people like knaves, out for anything they can get, might change their behaviour in undesirable ways. If people are given incentives to act in particular ways, they are more likely to do so – professionals will not do tasks for low payment which formerly they did for nothing.[24]

The argument that bureaucrats and politicians are self-interested has led public choice theorists to two different conclusions. The first has been the view that governments could not be reformed and that voters were at the mercy of public sector monopolies. This led to the argument that public sector monopolies need to be broken up, to allow for increased competition and therefore increase individual choice in the purchase of health or education. Privatisation of public services was a major pillar of reform advocated by public choice theorists. Privatisation, it was argued, would break up the knowledge estate of public sector professionals; it would encourage new entrants and therefore create competition in the supply of goods which would increase choice for the consumers.

Public choice theory is not the same as liberal market theory but it begins from the same assumptions, and there are important links between the theory and the arguments of liberals. Public choice theorists have argued for the need to create market disciplines in areas of government provision. The discipline of the market creates more choice for consumers, it creates accountability and transparency in public provision and it creates the discipline of the price mechanism. Public sector provision favours those who know their way around politics, those who have access to politicians, political parties, those who can lobby and those who join strategic interest groups. The context of public provision therefore acts against the interest of the individual. In this sense the argument is that the public sector is shaped by and is of benefit to those who work within it rather than the clients it seeks to serve. Poor performances in schools, hospital waiting lists, delayed payments of social security, fraud and inadequate accountability of public finances are all attributed to the problems of monopoly in the provision of public services.

Extending public choice can also be achieved through a process of reforming public sector institutions by establishing constitutions that make these institutions transparent, accountable and open to scrutiny. Governments can be made more transparent. Accountability to democratic procedures, open constitutions, judicial review and an independent central bank are also processes which provide a check and balance on politicians, bureaucracy and public sector professionals.

Liberalism and welfare

The position of liberals in relation to welfare is double-edged. On the one hand, liberalism favours universal human rights and opposes discrimination. On the other, liberals tend to view intervention by the state with considerable scepticism; the role of the state in welfare provision has to be confined to a minimum in order to protect individual liberty and avoid the abuses to which government activities are prone. The same strictures do not apply to all forms of welfare, because this does not apply to insurance, mutual aid, and voluntary forms of social protection – the dominant pattern in Europe. Although there are those on the right, particularly in the USA, who argue against redistribution and the production of dependency through social protection, the arguments are based in a central misapprehension – the belief that welfare is simply the product of compulsory intervention by the state. In many cases, it is not.

Privatisation has been an essential pillar of liberal policy. It is seen as extending choice to the individual, since privatisation is the means of breaking with public sector monopolies. Privatisation takes different forms including the contracting out of service, the denationalisation of public utilities, the liberalisation of the professions, deregulation of labour markets and removing artificial barriers to entry. Privatisation policy breaks with the monopoly of public sector trade unions and other sectional interests. The process of tendering and contracting out of services means that public sector unions are forced to compete in offering lower costs to win tenders. The costs of delivering a service is now made more transparent – the government is no longer the direct employer and wages are therefore contextualised within the market place.

The belief in the superiority of the market as a form of distribution has also been associated with the development of quasi-markets in the provision of public services.[25] Quasi-markets are an attempt to introduce the disciplines of the market into the provision of public services. They are developed by identifying suppliers and consumers of services which may be financed from the tax system and provided by government, but which then operate through the price mechanism. The state in this context no longer acts as the provider but as the enabler of the individual choice. The enabling role of the state is a way of shifting muscle power away from sectional interests to the citizen by making the consumer sovereign through the price mechanism. The consumer is sovereign when their competition and the consumer has the ability to pay. The ability to pay can be extended by giving the consumer tax incentives in the purchase of private health insurance, private pension plans and the provision of education vouchers in the purchase of education from local schools. The ability to pay creates the means of ensuring that schools, colleges, hospitals and doctors start to listen to their clients and provide services which their clients want rather than the service they want to provide.

Chapter 5

Conservatism and the New Right

The nature of conservatism

The idea of 'conservatism' stands for a wide range of very different approaches to politics. It embraces ideological traditionalists, political mystics, modern pragmatists and reformers – as well, for some, as the liberal individualism described in the previous chapter. There is a form of conservatism which is authoritarian and emphasises social order; there is a moral, religious voice, emphasising work, family and country; there is a conservatism which emphasises solidarity, integration, and social responsibility; and there is a conservatism which tries to avoid principles and proceed pragmatically. Some views run across different forms of conservative thought: they include the values of property and tradition, and an acceptance of inequalities. At the same time, there is a wide range of views considered here, and it is difficult to identify a single, consistent approach.

The values of feudal society

In feudal times, social relationships were characterised by a strongly hierarchical social structure, supported by moral values of religion, loyalty (which was both personal and political) and the dominance of status ascribed to a person at birth. In the words of a famous hymn,

> The rich man at his castle, the poor man at his gate
> God made them high and lowly, and ordered their estate.

The most extreme form of social stratification in the present day is found in a caste society, where marriage, work and personal status are conditioned by the caste into which a person is born; but there are many other residual elements of feudal relationships, including the respect accorded to people born to high status (like the Queen of England), the idea that the head of state is like the head of a family (still an important concept in South-east Asia), differentiation between people on the basis of 'race' (which is a form of caste) and the automatic acquisition of property rights by inheritance. In a feudal society, people of higher status required a level of protection appropriate to that status rather than to their need, and people of lower status needed less. There is a strong emphasis on social order and the importance of authority.

The defence of this kind of social system is associated with the political 'right', but it is a very different kind of right wing from the 'New Right' associated with liberal individualism. In parts of Europe, including in particular Spain and Italy, it has been associated with fascism; in the nineteenth century, it was identified with the reactionary politics of the 'ultras'; in some countries, including Greece and France, there is an association with authoritarian militarism. The tradition in the UK is identified with the 'Tories' (a term dominant in the eighteenth century, and now often used as a casual reference to the present-day Conservative Party, though their politics are very different).

The implications for welfare are complex. On the one hand, the stratification of society favoured in this model presents an important barrier to the protection of individuals, and the fundamental inequalities seem to offer little to those who are marginal or excluded. On the other, feudal values also argued for charity and the principle that *noblesse oblige*, that rich people must give to poor people. Resources in society were distributed according to status, so that those in the highest caste would receive treatment which was appropriate to that status, and those in the lowest would receive the least. (There is still in the UK an active 'Society for Distressed Gentlefolk'.) In other words, welfare would not be simply denied, but would be stratified, on the same principles as the rest of society. The 'conservative–corporatist' model of welfare applied in continental Europe – initiated by Bismarck, a member of the semi-feudal Junker class – reflects the principle to some degree: welfare is not universal, but stratified by occupation.

The organic society

A second important strand in conservative thought is the idea of society as an organic whole. Taken literally, the description of society as 'organic' suggests that it is somehow a living thing like a plant, and there have been thinkers who take that view quite seriously: analogies between society and the body have been commonplace. The medieval philosopher Marsiglio of Padua, himself a physician, wrote about political community in terms of the health and disease of the community.[1] Bradley, an English nineteenth-century philosopher whose view of the state sometimes verged on the metaphysical, argued for 'social surgery' to cut out the diseased elements of society.[2]

Modern conservatives have tended to take the idea of organic relations rather less literally. The organic view of society is one based on the existence of complex, overlapping networks, relationships which are so varied and manifold that they defy any simple description. The arguments used by some liberals, like Spencer or Hayek, overlap with this view: both argued that society was so complex, and the relationships so convoluted, that it is impossible meaningfully to intervene in social relationships without producing undesired, unintended consequences.

The view of society as a complex network of social relationships is most clearly compatible with schemes of welfare based on occupational record, contribution and membership of a particular community. But it is difficult to see the organic view of society as having any simple, clearly identifiable implication for welfare; the difference between social surgery on the one hand, or non-intervention on the other, is enormous.

Moral principles

The nature of the social structure in feudal society was bound by duties, primarily religious in nature, and many aristocrats acted as patricians – superior beings with a moral obligation to the lesser orders. In Britain, this was the view of the 'Old Whigs' who opposed the Tories;[3] it extended into the management of the colonies, where Kipling enjoined the English to 'take up the white man's burden'. This approach is still visible in some missionary work in developing countries.

In the present day, these ideas have been gradually transmuted into a powerful moral view of society. Often it is informed by religious belief: in Europe it is identified with the idea of Christian Democracy. The values of work, family and country, frequently emphasised by the political right, are all cases in which positive moral duties are encouraged. At the same time, morality implies restrictions and constraints on actions – most obviously in relation to abortion, because that is a prominent moral issue, but also affecting views of crime and family matters like divorce.

Solidarity and one-nation conservatism

A fourth strand of conservative thought rests in the idea of moral responsibility. Duties and obligations, rather than rights, are the root of social relationships. Conservatism of this kind is informed not simply by moral values, but a strong sense of social responsibility. Social Catholicism, in particular, argues that society is based in a set of moral obligations, and that people are part of a system of social networks in which they have mutual responsibilities to each other.[4] This implies a commitment to co-operation, and indeed to some level of redistribution to ensure that people are not excluded from social contact.

In the UK, this kind of moral commitment to those who are excluded is most closely identified with the 'one-nation' conservatism espoused by Disraeli. This stems from a different tradition, and the rationale is accordingly different: the idea of one nation rests partly in moral obligations to others, but also partly in the value of the nation itself. One-nation conservatives argued for a 'property-owning democracy', giving people a 'stake in the country' by ensuring that they had ownership of property and were able to participate in economic processes. But there is an important difference between this approach and the solidarity favoured by Christian Democrats in Europe. Solidarity, in Christian Democracy, implies mutual aid and social protection; one-nation conservatism was concerned less with protection, and more with economic integration.

Pragmatism

The defenders of feudal values were opposed in their day by two very different kinds of political view. One, held by the liberals, became the main substantive opposition; liberal individualism denied the central moral legitimacy of the social structure. The other important view was that of the pragmatists, who were not interested in ideological nostrums and wanted a form of government which made life better. This was the view of the 'new Whigs', most famously represented by Lord Halifax, whose *Character of a Trimmer* defended the practice of adjusting to political circumstances as circumstances demanded,[5] and Edmund Burke. Burke supported the American Revolution, and opposed the French: while he accepted that the American colonists had a reasonable argument, he reacted strongly against the attempts of the French Revolutionists to reform everything, including community, science, religion and the calendar. 'The science of constructing a commonwealth, or renovating it, or reforming it, is not, like any other experimental science, to be performed a priori.'[6] Burke defended tradition, but he did not defend every part of it. Things change, and the practice of government had to change with them. 'A state without the means of change is without the means of its conservation.'[7] He argued that many things were the way they were for a good reason, even if it was sometimes difficult to see. Radical change led to radical mistakes. The way to go about reforming society was a little at a time, in slow, incremental steps, finding out what worked and rejecting what did not. Burke is often described as the father of the English Conservative Party; he was also described by Richard Crossman, without irony, as the father of the Labour Party.

The conservative tradition is seen by many commentators as fundamentally non-ideological – a position hotly disputed by sociologists who argue, after Mannheim, that ideology is inescapable.[8] The basis of the conservative position is scepticism: the belief that preconceived ideals, concepts and principles cannot be trusted, and have the potential to be dangerous. This is sometimes coupled with scepticism about human nature – that the people who propose the grand ideas should not be trusted either. The test of what was appropriate was to try it on the small scale, and see if it worked.

Conservatism and the state

There is no simple position on welfare which can be identified as conservative. Authoritarianism, moral values, social responsibility and pragmatism do not always sit very comfortably together – though of course they may do. To complicate issues further, conservatism is frequently aligned in European politics with liberalism, because it can be used to defend property rights. But there are clear tensions between authoritarianism and individual rights, political liberalism and the defence of social status, social responsibility and *laissez-faire*.

Conservatives are not, in general, averse to state intervention: the views considered here include a strong emphasis on law and order, a concern with moral intervention and a pragmatic willingness to use intervention to do whatever is appropriate in the circumstances. Conservatism is sometimes represented as the 'politics of power', sometimes as the 'art of statecraft', a willingness to use and manage the affairs of government to meet socially desired ends.

At the same time, there are also elements in conservative thought which are sceptical about the role of government, and which argue for restriction in its power and authority. The importance of religious principles, the influence of liberal thought and the concern to protect what is valuable in social relationships all imply limitations on the scope of state activity. In Europe, these limitations are often discussed in terms of 'subsidiarity'.

The concept of subsidiarity emerged in Catholic teaching in the nineteenth century, but the classic statement of subsidiarity in Catholic social teaching was made by Pius XI in *Quadragesimo Anno* in 1931. The encyclical suggests that 'it is wrong to withdraw from the individual and to commit to the community at large what private enterprise and endeavour can accomplish'.[9] This is individualistic, restricting the power of the state, and it has attracted support from liberals on the right.

The argument continues, however, with some important qualifications. The second main point in the encyclical's definition of subsidiarity is that 'it is likewise unjust and a gravely harmful disturbance of right order to turn over to a greater society of higher rank functions and services which can be performed by lesser bodies on a lower plane'.[10] This is decentralist; power should be devolved to the lowest level possible. The European Commission argues that subsidiarity means 'that decisions are taken as close as possible to the citizen',[11] and the argument for decentralisation can be seen in the case for a 'Europe of the Regions'.

The third main point is that collective bodies have a responsibility to aid and assist lower bodies: 'for a social undertaking of any sort, by its very nature, ought to aid the members of the body social, but never to destroy and absorb them'.[12] This qualifies the first principle;

the idea of subsidiarity is not unequivocally opposed to the state. Rather, it establishes the conditions for the state's role. Jacques Delors, formerly president of the European Commission, has argued:

> Subsidiarity is not only a limit to the intervention of a higher authority in relation to a person or a collectivity which is able to act itself, it is also an obligation to act in relation to this person or this collectivity to offer the means to accomplish their aims.[13]

This is largely consistent with the Catholic concept.

The fourth point relates not so much to the explicit terms in which subsidiarity is defined as to its implicit role in Catholic social teaching. The principle relates not only to the state and society but is also concerned with defining the role of the Church in that society; restricting the role of the state has the effect of reserving to the Church a number of functions, for example in health and social care, which in other circumstances may fall within the remit of the state. The Catholic Church is not, however, a structure in which authority is decentralised; what it does is define a series of universal principles which may be implemented differently in different social contexts. In Italy, Cardinal Casaroli, a former Vatican secretary of state, has attacked proposed Community legislation on issues like abortion as 'a violation of subsidiarity and of the Church's authority'.[14]

Subsidiarity is not the only way in which reservations are expressed, and it may be helpful to consider an alternative concept, developed in the Netherlands: the idea of 'sphere sovereignty'. This idea was developed in the Dutch Anti-Revolutionary Party in the nineteenth century, as a means of expressing the views of Calvinist Christians on state intervention. Sphere sovereignty refers to the independence of different groups in social and economic life. Kuyper wrote:

> In a Calvinistic sense, we understand hereby, that the family, the business, science, art and so forth are all social spheres, which do not owe their existence to the state, and which do not derive the law of their life from the superiority of the state, but obey a high authority within their own bosom;

an authority which rules, by the grace of God, just as the sovereignty of the State does.[15]

Kuyper attributed the independence of the spheres to God: 'all together they form the life of creation, in accord with the ordinances of creation, and therefore are organically developed.'[16] The spheres were, then, to be literally sacrosanct. One important aspect in which sphere sovereignty and subsidiarity overlap is in their concern to maintain an independent role for the Church in relation to the state. Dooyeweerd's influential expression of the doctrine tends somewhat to blur the lines of division; the state is given a legitimate role in regulating actions which allows, for example, for intervention in cases of domestic violence.[17] However, it seems clear that the idea of sphere sovereignty does entail a presumption of non-interference. It lies at the root of the 'pillarisation' of Dutch society, which offered a high degree of autonomy to Catholic, Protestant and secular branches of society.[18] Although the connection is indirect, this philosophy also played a part in the justification of South African apartheid.

Both positions limit the scope and legitimacy of state intervention. There is an important difference between subsidiarity and sphere sovereignty. Subsidiarity recognises the legitimacy of state action: sphere sovereignty tends to assume that intervention in social spheres is illegitimate. However, when the Dutch right-wing Catholic and Protestant parties merged in the 1980s, to form the new Christian Democratic Party, they agreed that there was no fundamental difference in their positions.

The New Right

Conservatism has enjoyed a intellectual revival in recent years. The new conservatism reflects three layers of interest: moral, political and economic.

The Moral New Right

The central theme of this approach is that there is such a thing as society and that there are some core elements which hold society together but which have been undermined by liberalism. The Moral New Right argument is that welfare states have acted as a moral hazard which has undermined the ethics of responsibility, caring and solidarity. Welfare states financed through the tax system encouraged a feeling that the state would take the responsibility of caring which was the domain of the family (for the family read women). Because people paid taxes they shifted responsibility to the caring professionals, including doctors, teachers, nurses and social workers – the do-gooders of the 1960s. The moral argument is that authority, tradition and institutions which had previously acted as the glue which held society institutions have all been undermined. The welfare state with its plethora of family benefits has encouraged the break-up of families because it has made it more viable for women to choose to leave family settings and as single parents to bring up children. Teenage crime and violence is blamed on the absence of fathers to act as role models for growing-up boys.

The Moral New Right is organicist – it emphasises the practices that hold communities and families together, including religion, political elites and traditional institutions. It is these settings which give the individual a sense of identity, belonging and anchoring within a community setting. The Moral New Right therefore emphasises social responsibility, giving and the common good rather than citizenship, the individual and individual rights.

The major dilemma for the Moral New Right is the market economy. If the major concern is to recreate a specific sense of belonging, to recreate the community, setting the support for the market economy seems to be a contradiction. The dynamics of the market have unhinged and undermined many industrial communities, as those communities were deemed as no longer economically viable and they were priced out of the labour market. The market economy has contributed to the making of strangers as communities break up and individuals go to seek employment in new settings.

According to this perspective the aim is to generate a greater sense of personal responsibility – where individuals take responsibility for their actions so that those involved in crime take responsibility for their actions and therefore are punished accordingly. Individuals are part of their communities and are therefore responsible to their community in the process of giving and caring for others. The 'active citizen' involved in voluntary and charity work is an important element in the creating of a moral community. The Moral New Right seeks therefore to remoralise the family by advocating more stringent rules on divorce, making fathers more accountable for their children and removing welfare entitlements for single mothers. The Moral New Right tends to point out that the welfare state has encouraged the increase in numbers of single mothers through housing and social security payments.

The welfare state is replaced by welfare society where the voluntary sector, charities, government and the commercial sector become essential components of welfare society. The moral hazard encouraged by a welfare state which encouraged rights over responsibility and limited the sense of responsibility to the paying of taxes is replaced by a sense of belonging, solidarity and identity within the practices of community.

The Political New Right

The Political New Right points to the decline of politics, with voters becoming increasingly disenchanted with the established political parties, the corruption of public spaces and democracy reflecting a series of broken promises. The Political New Right seeks to replace politics from being a contract between electors and government to a politics which is founded on allegiance, authority and a respect for public institutions. The commitment of allegiance suggests that people's commitment to democracy should be founded on trust and hope in the government they elect rather than on narrow accountancy issues of taxation and public expenditure.

The Political New Right puts an emphasis on the importance of the symbols in public life including the monarchy in the UK, and the Presidency in France and the USA. All these institutions are perceived as symbols of nationhood and national identity.

The Economic New Right

The economics of the New Right is the economics of market liberalism, marked by a commitment to the concepts of rational agency, the price mechanism and competitive markets. In contrast to the Moral and Political New Right, the economic New Right places greater emphasis on rational individualism, the individual who acts in self-interest, the individual who should be the end rather than the means to an end. The individual is therefore unencumbered rather than encumbered in community or national settings.

The major criticism by the Economic New Right of the welfare state is that the welfare state is coercive: it removes the individual's right to choose and reduces the freedom of the individual through the tax system. The welfare state sets the priorities of how income should be spent rather than allowing individuals to make their own priorities.

At the macro-economic level the Economic New Right points to the problems of inflation brought about by too much government borrowing and the reluctance of government to finance welfare expenditures through taxation. The welfare state crowds out the private sector both in terms of finance and resources. Financial crowding out is attributed to government borrowing and the need therefore to increase interest rates. Higher interest rates push up the costs of investment and therefore deter companies from borrowing because of the higher costs. The government crowds out the private sector in terms of resources because as government employment increases, there is an increase in the demand of labour, which in turn pushes up wage costs.

The Economic New Right is associated with monetarist thinking in the making of economic policy. According to this approach, the priority of government is the control of inflation which means the control of the money supply and government borrowing. Because individuals are rational agents, governments can only succeed to reduce inflation by making explicit their macro-economic policy. Agents bargaining for wages do so in the knowledge that the government is committed to the control of inflation, so that wage bargains do not have to include future inflation expectations.

The economics of the New Right is also associated with the thinking of supply-side economics. The approach of the supply siders is that the solution to unemployment is mainly to be found in improving the flexibility of labour supply so that the cost of labour will fall and increase demand. The supply siders point to rigidities in the labour market, including the role of trade unions and their influence in restricting the numbers entering specific labour markets through artificial barriers on recruitment, training and restrictive practices. Trade union reform and removing trade union immunities is therefore essential to removing a major obstacle in the supply of labour.

Supply siders also point to the impact of social security on employment arguing that the social security system prolongs unemployment duration because workers can rely on social security in moving between jobs. Supply siders would therefore argue that unemployment is voluntary and that if government is committed to reducing the rate of unemployment they also have to reduce the level of benefits so that benefits became less of an incentive.

Reducing the levels of benefits, taxing benefit, putting limits on eligibility are policies that would improve labour supply.

Supply siders would also favour the reduction of taxation rather than the increase in public expenditure. Reducing personal taxes creates incentives for individuals to work since the rewards of work now benefit the individual directly rather than the government. A tax reduction is similar to a wage increase since a reduction in taxes results in an increase in take-home pay, which in turn increases household income and therefore demand for goods and services. By contrast, an increase in tax to finance higher levels of public expenditure is seen as a reduction in take-home pay, and employees seek to redress the tax increase by pushing up their wage demands. This, in turn, results in inflation and job losses. The tax reduction, by contrast, reduces the pressures on wage inflation and therefore workers are less likely to price themselves out of the labour market.

Within the context of the economics of the New Right, the primary aim is to create a climate of flexible and deregulated labour markets, with minimum government intervention in the setting of wages or conditions of work, employment rights or duration of hours worked. Wages reflect the marginal product of labour and any attempt to increase the wage beyond the marginal product is likely to result in unemployment. New Right economists are opposed to intervention in the dynamics of the labour market. They would prefer negative income tax and government payments to the employed to deal with problems of poverty and wage inequality.

The new conservatism

Although these three approaches represent very different schools of thought, they have important elements in common. The home domain is their criticism of big government, the welfare state and the liberal establishment, including the economics of Keynes, the new public sector professionals and collectivist values. The New Right argues for the reduction of the role of government in the provision of welfare services, substituting individual responsibility and individual choice. The control of inflation is the primary issue in the conduct of economic policy; the New Right argues that government and public sector deficits have devalued the currency. The objection to intervention is not straightforward. Part is liberal; part may be seen as pluralist, in the sense that intervention which is permissible in one sphere may not be accepted in another; and part is pragmatic, based on the view that some forms of intervention are established and work, while others are not established or do not. At the same time, a number of conservative arguments point towards intervention: emphasis on the value of the family, a stress on social order, a concern with heritage. Despite the emphasis in some quarters on a minimal state, few conservatives or liberals are actively opposed to the state being involved in, for example, education or conservation. The Christian Democratic approach in western Europe goes further, arguing for moral intervention, a recognition of social responsibility (or solidarity) and a stress on social cohesion.

Although there are areas of agreement, the New Right also reflects a series of tensions and contradictions. The Economic New Right argues that the individual is rational and is capable of making decisions and that therefore market exchanges should be seen as the moral transactions between competent individuals. By contrast, the Moral New Right favours a state which is highly moralistic, which seeks to cement society together through ethics of responsibility, allegiance, authority and tradition. The Moral New Right points to the primacy of community and the situated individual within community settings; the market liberal puts the emphasis on the individual, on individual life projects. Market liberals might argue that drug abuse should be decriminalised and that drugs should be left to the market, where the role of the state is limited to providing information about health and thus respecting the rights of the individual. The Moral New Right wants to protect the individual and society and therefore seeks to prohibit the use/ abuse of drugs because, they argue, individuals cannot be trusted to make decisions. The Moral New Right has specific views on pornography, the use of the internet and the family. The Economic New Right seeks to resist any attempt to moralise for the good society but instead favours the role of the marketplace as being the place where individuals decide their priorities.

Much of the development of the new conservatism has been based in an unlikely fusion of liberalism with the ideas reviewed in this chapter – unlikely because there are tensions and contradictions between individualism and a stratified society, the ideological nature of libertarianism and the practicality of conservatism, the emphasis on the free market and the value attached to social order. The New Right uses individualistic arguments in relation to the market, but often uses conservative arguments when considering social relationships, like the position of the family or the importance of social order. It does not seem to matter very much that the positions are based in different intellectual premises, or that they conflict in practice, because they are consistent in another way: both are used to support an idealised status quo, to resist people who argue for social change, and most importantly to object to intervention by government or the state.

Chapter 6

Social democracy and socialism

Social democracy

Social democracy is not a system of ideas, but rather a set of principles and values which some people apply to the political process. There are two essential principles. First, social democracy is 'democratic'; second, it is 'social'.

Democracy is a form of government in which authority is derived from the people who are governed. This term is much abused – there is hardly a government in the world which would not claim to be democratic, in the sense of having some authority derived from the people who are governed. It says very little to state that a government has been elected: many elections, and possibly most, are coerced, corrupt, or confined to one party. A government with authority derived from the people may still be oppressive and undemocratic – the most notorious example is the German National Socialist government, elected through a legitimate procedure in 1933.

The western model of democracy, to which social democrats generally refer, is commonly referred to as 'liberal democracy'. It is characterised not simply by the process of election but by a system of values, based on protection for the rights of individuals and minorities. The emphasis on rights is linked to the processes of democracy not just by historical accident, but because democratic thinkers (especially James Madison, one of the framers of the American constitution)[1] argued that protection of minority interests was fundamental to legitimate decision-making. The basis of majority decision-making in the American constitution was that each majority was made up of shifting coalitions of different minority groups. It was important both to ensure that power was never vested in the hands of a consistent majority, and to protect the situation of individuals when majority decisions were made. The essential element of liberal democracy is not, then, rule by the people, but the establishment of procedures and rights which protect the situation of the people who are ruled.

The 'social' element of social democracy is based in collective action, which can be understood either as mutual aid or as action with a common purpose. Mutual aid is expressed through a network of rights and responsibilities in society; characteristic examples include both informal networks of family and community, and formal arrangements such as occupational welfare and friendly societies (or 'mutualities'). Action with a common purpose, or joint action, is commonly favoured in the form of collaborative or co-operative arrangements. Owenism, an approach taken by an enlightened employer in the early days of the Industrial Revolution, argued for collaboration of workers and employers, and promotion of the welfare of employees.[2] This had some influence on the labour movement in Britain and the USA. In France, there is considerable emphasis on the role of industry and labour as 'social partners', and the formal mechanisms of welfare attempt to balance and represent the interests of the different factions. In continental Europe, this kind of approach is often linked with 'corporatism', in which the state attempts to co-ordinate and foster collaboration between different interest groups. Corporatism can be seen as an attempt to control the different factions, but it can also be seen as a system for ensuring the representation of their interests and promoting collaborative effort.

Social democracy combines elements of individualism and collectivism: it is liable to be individualistic in the defence of rights, and collectivist in the development of government action and intervention. The balance can be struck in different ways, and people who have described themselves as social democrats may appear to be left- or right-wing in different contexts. The primary opposition to social democracy comes, on the one hand, from liberals and the 'New Right', who believe that the acceptance of collectivist premises and state intervention is dangerous to individual rights, and on the other from socialists who are concerned that the principles of social democracy are liable to be undermined by social inequality.

Social democracy and the market

Markets represent, at least in theory, the result of the interactions of individuals, who are involved in producing, trading or obtaining things for consumption. Although this is held by some individualists, and particularly by the New Right, to lead to the best possible distribution of resources, there are some clear cases of 'market failure', in which markets fail to deliver. Some markets, like agricultural markets, tend to be unstable, and without intervention this may lead to hardship or even collapse. There are problems when the effect of transactions between some people affect others – the issue of 'externalities'. Pollution, for example, is a negative externality; training for work undertaken in the education system is a positive externality. Some things are public goods, like roads or street lighting, because the benefit to the public in general is greater than to any single user, and markets have generally failed to provide them.

The other main problem with markets is that they do not guarantee the welfare of everyone. Some people are excluded: there is generally some form of 'adverse selection', in which people who are difficult to provide for are left out. (This can happen, for example, because of high levels of need, because of relatively low incomes, and because of location – it may not be economic to provide services to people who live on remote islands or on mountain sides.) There are also cases of 'diswelfare', where people are adversely affected by the actions of other people in the market. People may be selected out of the labour market, for example, because of physical limitations like disability, or outmoded skills. If the aim is to provide services for all – as a matter of citizenship or rights – some form of intervention, and perhaps some form of compensatory mechanism, is required.

Social democrats, because they accept a number of individualist premises, are also likely to accept the principle of the market. However, where there are social objectives to be met, or where markets fail, there may be a case for some degree of intervention. On that basis, social democrats tend to favour a mixed economy – an economy in which some activities will be undertaken on a collective basis, while others will be left to individuals.

Citizenship and social rights

In the period since the Second World War, social democracy has been strongly associated with the development of the European welfare states. The connection is not a firm one, because other kinds of political belief can also be used in support of the provision of welfare, but social democracy can be taken as explicit justification for the kind of welfare state which actually exists – based in political democracy and a mixed economy. T. H. Marshall, in a famous analysis, argued that the right to welfare was closely linked to democracy. Rights were both the outcome of the democratic process, and necessary for someone to be able to participate in society.[3]

The emphasis on political and economic rights which had characterised the politics of the eighteenth and nineteenth century had been supplemented in the twentieth century by social rights. Marshall wrote of the 'right to welfare', which refers to a general status rather than a specific form of right. Another way of expressing this was the term 'citizenship', defined by as 'a status bestowed on those who are full members of a community. All those who possess the status are equal with respect to the rights and duties with which the status is endowed.'[4] In the political sense, citizenship refers to membership of a political community, generally implying rights including rights of residence and a legal status, and responsibilities including subjection to the law of that community. Marshall extended the idea of citizenship to refer to the social rights associated with welfare, and the idea of citizenship has been used to refer to a general and inclusive status in which all people will have a right to receive social and public service.

Giddens has criticised Marshall for providing an approach which seems to be 'evolutionary', an argument which seems to depend on an inevitable logic. This interpretation of Marshall can be challenged.[5] Marshall suggests that rights which had existed in the seventeenth and eighteenth century had been eroded in the nineteenth century to be revived in the twentieth century. His approach is based on contingency and political choice, on struggles and on the ebbs and flows of these struggles.

Citizenship has meant reciprocity of rights and duties within the community, membership of the community and participation. Citizenship is not something inherent in each person, but a status, and it may be conditional on some form of qualification. This inevitably involves some contest about who is, and who is not, a citizen.

Citizenship has often been held to be contingent, for example, on contribution to society, civic competence or independence. Because citizenship is a status which people may or may not have, there cannot be a presumption of equality between citizens and non-citizens – indeed, such equality would make nonsense of the idea, because if the idea of citizenship means anything, it is that people will be treated differently as a result of having it. If the right to welfare is based on membership of a community, there must be those who are not considered members, and so who are not citizens. Often, they are people of different races, different nationalities, or (as in much of Europe) migrant workers.

The idea of citizenship has, then, important limitations. A concept which is based in membership necessarily defines an out-group – those who are not citizens – as well as the in-group of those who are. Citizenship does not imply universal coverage unless citizenship itself is universal, and it is the nature of citizenship that some people are liable to be left out. This may include, for example, children (who are not accepted as citizens until they come of age, and whose rights are often contingent on the status of their parents), immigrants (who are not members of the community until the status of citizenship is awarded), and convicts (who may be held in some circumstances to have sacrificed their basic rights; although most people in western society would agree that slavery is illegitimate, people in prison are still subject to forced labour). The concept of citizenship may also be used to exclude some people, like those with mental illness or severe learning disabilities, whose membership of society is treated as defeasible.

Although the idea of citizenship and the right to welfare were linked in the UK with 'universality', or application to everyone, the term is something of a misnomer. The development of citizenship in the post-war period has been characterised not so much by the spread of universal citizenship as by a process of generalisation. Over time, social rights have been progressively extended to include more and more people. In continental Europe, this has often been done through the extension of particular rather than general rights. General rights are rights which apply to everyone; particular rights apply to individuals in specific circumstances, for example as the result of a contract or as compensation for personal injury. Rights to welfare in much of Europe are particular; they are earned through specific contributions and directly related to each person's work record. A person who retires in France or Germany will have a pension, often made up from a range of sources, based on contributions to different funds over the years. In principle, this implies a considerable potential to be left out, and this has been a major problem in both countries; the German response has been to try to maximise economic activity, and so participation in the labour market, while France has emphasised the progressive extension of pension arrangements and the intervention of the state in balancing contributions and funds. Social democracy is not then necessarily linked to equality of status for all; people have a right to welfare, but it does not mean that they will have the same access to services or an equivalent standard of welfare.

Another way of describing this pattern of provision is the concept of 'institutional welfare', originally proposed by Wilensky and Lebeaux to describe a society in which the provision of welfare would be an accepted and normal part of social life.[6] Certain needs, like the needs of childhood, old age, sickness and (possibly) unemployment, are needs which potentially affect anyone, and which are defined and generated by the society in which a person lives. They are, in that sense, 'institutional' needs – needs which are built into the fabric of society – and they require a general institutional response. The term is most clearly associated with the postwar ideal of the welfare state in the UK, though some other societies (like Sweden) have been represented as having institutional welfare states.

Institutional welfare is linked to the arguments of social democracy partly by historical accident – it happened that the democratic countries in which welfare is socially accepted have been described as institutional, while others in Eastern Europe which sought to develop· provision for welfare were not – but also because there is a conceptual link. The model of institutional welfare helps to define the 'social' or collective element of social democracy. Although some writers have associated institutional welfare with particular views – Titmuss thinks of it as redistributive or egalitarian,[7] while Mishra takes it to relate to a mixed economy and partial coverage[8] – the position is more simply that the nature of institutional welfare is indeterminate; the idea that needs and services are 'normal' says very little about the shape and format that the services will take, except that they will not be confined to a narrow section of the population and will not be accompanied by the penalties and loss of status which are associated with residual provision. In the context of the discussion of social democracy, the key elements in institutional welfare are the views that there should be general arrangements for commonly occurring needs; that arrangements for welfare will be collectively organised (for example, by the state or by mutualist societies) rather than commercially based; and that they will be provided without imposing or threatening a loss of citizenship. Despite many differences, these modest aims are fairly generally accepted in the countries of the European Union.

Socialism

There are many different kinds of socialist belief; they range from Marxist and quasi-Marxist analyses on one hand to some beliefs which might better be described as social democracy. Like social democracy, socialism is not a doctrine or ideology so much as a set of principles which are applied differently in different contexts.

The key principles are the principles of the French Revolution: liberty, equality and fraternity. These issues have sometimes been interpreted individualistically, but in socialism they are generally presented in collective, social terms. To an individualist, freedom consists of the autonomy of the individual – the ability of each person to make decisions, to avoid constraints and to act. Equality consists of treatment as an equal, so that people should not be subject to discrimination. Fraternity means that individuals are able to co-operate with others, and to make arrangements with them for their mutual benefit. To a collectivist, freedom depends on the social environment, and personal ends are often achieved through joint action with others. Equality may be concerned with treatment as an equal, but substantive equality calls for a fair distribution of resources, which often means the elimination of disadvantage in outcomes. Fraternity is seen in terms of social cohesion and group action. Social democracy is liable to be individualistic, or to combine elements of individualism and collectivism; socialism is liable to be collectivist, leading to a different emphasis and a different interpretation of key principles. Where there are social problems, such as crime, drug abuse, poverty or homelessness, socialists look to social factors – the collective structures which foster these problems – rather than individual pathology. Where there are possible responses, socialists consider changes in social organisation and relationships rather than the behaviour of the individual. This does not mean that socialists ignore individual elements; on the contrary, there is a strong moral tradition in socialism based on each person's reponsibility to others and to society. But there is general scepticism about the liberal belief that people can avoid unemployment by individual effort, or that raising children is solely a matter for the parents. A wider society creates the conditions in which these circumstances apply and their consequences affect a wider society, not just the individuals involved.

The interpretation of liberty, equality and fraternity in socialist thought depends crucially on this collectivist approach. Freedom has been described as 'triadic', having three elements; to be free, a *person* must be free *from* restraint *to do* something.[9] A social view of freedom understands freedom mainly as a relationship between people; what people are able to do depends both on their own ability to act, and on the actions of others around them. 'Freedom', Tawney wrote, 'is always relative to power'.[10] People who are homeless, disabled, or unemployed are constrained by their circumstances, and by the effect of their circumstances on their relations with other people; they lack power, and their freedom is limited.

The objective of equality is particularly important to socialism – not least because it is the strongest distinction between socialism and social democratic thought. Relatively few people nowadays are opposed to equality in all its aspects; the idea that people should be treated as equals, without discrimination or favour by reason of birth, is accepted as much by the liberals of the New Right as by the left. The main difference relates to the application of the principle of equality in different circumstances. The question, Tawney argues, is how far the movement towards equality should be carried forward.[11] Socialists argue for equality not simply in procedures but in the distribution of resources, and not just in starting positions but in outcomes.

The issue of equality is often misrepresented in the literature, and since it is fundamental to an understanding of socialism, it is important to clarify it here. To say that people should be equal is not to say that they should be the same. Inequality consists not in difference, but in social disadvantage; equality is the removal of disadvantage. Equality between the sexes does not mean that men and women should be the same; the demand for gender equality is a demand for the removal of disadvantage. People might indeed be unequal as a result of physical characteristics, but the point of equality is not to change those characteristics; it is to eliminate the disadvantage. This is a general principle, rather than a specific pre-scription for action, and can be interpreted in a number of ways.[12] The kind of disadvantage which is being addressed might refer to individuals, to groups of people (for example, making women more equal or men) or to specific segments of society (for example, bring-ing poor pensioners nearer to rich pensioners). Many conflicts between socialists arise because some are concerned about one kind of equality (for example, inequality relating to race) while others are concerned with other kinds (for example, between rich and poor).

Some critics object to the elimination of disadvantage, because they believe that disadvantage can arise legitimately. Robert Nozick, for example, gives the example of a sports star who becomes rich because lots of people want to see him play and pay for the privilege. He argues that if people begin in a legitimate position, and the distribution of resources changes through a legitimate process, then the end result must also be legitimate. He objects to 'patterned' arguments about social justice, which try to impose a test on out-comes, as illegitimate.[13] The socialist demand for equality is based precisely in a judgment about outcomes. If the outcome of Nozick's legitimate distribution of resources is that some people go hungry while others have too much food, socialists argue for a redistribution of resources. (It is easier to justify this redistribution, of course, if one also thinks that the initial distribution is illegitimate, and many socialists do think so, but that is not necessary to the argu-ment.) In other words, socialism involves the imposition of moral judgments on the issues of distribution and disadvantage.

The interpretation of fraternity, similarly, tends to be strongly moralistic. Some socialist movements have been based around a general concept like the 'brotherhood of man' (important in the nineteenth century for the Independent Labour Party in Britain), while others, like 'guild socialists' and trades unionists, have been more narrowly focused on the solidarity of people in the workplace. Solidarity is generally expressed in two main ways: through the development of mechanisms of mutual aid and support, and through a generalised responsibility for other members of a society.[14] Society is linked – as it is in conservative thought – through a network of moral obligations.

Some aspects of socialist thought are strongly moralistic in their origins and expressions. Christian Socialism, for example, is based in a condemnation of the ethics of the market society and an emphasis on the responsibilities which people have to each other. The dissident tradition, based in Protestant thought, emphasised community and condemned the immorality of luxury and privilege. There is a strong utopian tradition linking ideas of altruism and membership of a human family. Other socialist beliefs emphasised a combination of moral principles along with practical benefits. The anti-commercialism of William Morris's Arts and Crafts movement combined a condemnation of the evils of modern industry with a utopian view of nature and society. Fabianism characteristically argued that collective action was both morally superior to the market and yielded greater benefits. (A classic example is Titmuss's book on the gift relationship, which claims to show both that the donation of blood is more moral and that it produces better-quality blood than the market does.[15]) The view of socialism as a moral doctrine is the key to understanding how many different strands of socialist thought have come together.

Socialism and the market

Two issues have distanced socialists from social democrats in the acceptance of the market. One is the historical link of socialism and the trades unions. In so far as capital and labour have been seen as antagonistic, socialism has been identified with the labour movement. This connection is outmoded to some degree, because many of the issues with which socialists are concerned cannot be represented in these terms. However, the 'social' is still associated in many countries with the issues of industrial relations and the collective organisation of working-class interests. Although there are countries in which the role of the trades unions has been relatively limited – notably Britain and the USA, where their role has tended to be confined to the industrial sphere – trades unions elsewhere have played a large part in the development of social policy, and in some European countries are responsible for the administration of social security benefits, housing and health services. The effect has been to reinforce the identification of socialism with collective organisation and mutual aid as an alternative to distribution through the market or reliance on employers.

More fundamentally, socialism is distanced from the market by its moral stance. Socialists judge the processes and outcomes of the market by the moral criteria which are applied to all issues of distribution and disadvantage. They have no particular predisposition against the market, but they have no predisposition for it either, and see no reason why they should accept its distributive consequences. This leads to an uneasy relationship: many socialists accept the existence of the market, and many of its consequences, without any conviction in its efficacy or fairness. In practice, few socialists are wholly opposed to the market in every respect; no one has seriously argued, for example, for a National Food Service (which is not intrinsically ridiculous – the UK government had substantial control over food production and distribution in the immediate post-war period, when the welfare state was founded). The main issue is to ensure that people have a fair share of resources, which means that they are later able to spend them on what they want. Opposition to the market is strongest in the areas in which it has been shown to fail, or where better alternatives have been demonstrated – for example, in the supply of water, brought under state control in Britain in the nineteenth century, or the supply of health care, in which collective systems are more economical and more universal.

Socialism and welfare

There is nothing intrinsically socialist about welfare provision; welfare provision has to be judged by the same moral criteria as other distributive mechanisms, and there are circumstances in which welfare provision may be discriminatory or inegalitarian. In general, though, socialists tend to emphasise the importance of welfare as a mechanism of redistribution. All social services are redistributive, in the sense that those who pay are different from those who receive. Socialists are concerned that this redistribution should be both progressive, which implies that richer people should pay more than poorer people, and egalitarian.

This also seems to imply that money should be taken from richer people and moved to poorer ones, but the situation is more complex than this; giving money to poorer people is a form of selectivity, and selectivity can be socially divisive, putting the recipients of poor relief in a social position where they are liable to be criticised and socially rejected. Tawney argued for a different approach. Public spending on social services was the most effective way of redistributing resources. The aim, he wrote, is not the division of the nation's income into eleven million fragments, to be distributed, without further ado, like cake at a school treat, among its eleven million families. It is, on the contrary, the pooling of its surplus resources by means of taxation, and the use of the funds thus obtained to make accessible to all, irrespective of their income, occupation or social position, the conditions of civilisation which, in the absence of such measures, can only be enjoyed by the rich.[16]

Julian Le Grand argues against this that the universal social services are not available equally to all. There is a general trend for universal social services, particularly in health and education, to favour the middle classes; other subsidies in transport and housing have a similar effect. On this basis, he suggests that the 'strategy of equality' proposed by Tawney has failed.[17] In an important respect, though, Le Grand misses the point. The issue is not whether middle-class people get a greater financial benefit, but the accessibility of social services to people who are disadvantaged, and the distributive consequences of public provision. The benefits to poorer people include not only what they actually receive, but the value of coverage (which in countries without comparable systems has to be paid for). On that basis, the effect of public provision appears to be substantially more egalitarian than Le Grand gives it credit for.

For some socialists, a concern with equality would not be enough to establish the legitimacy of welfare services. There are two other important criteria: liberty and fraternity. Freedom, or autonomy, is fostered partly by removing restrictions, and also by a process of empowerment, ensuring that people have the capacity to act. The arguments about empowerment are currently prominent in the discourse of social work, but they have always been a major part of discussions of education, and for many years socialists argued for educational provision as a primary means of realising socialist principles. The concern with solidarity has led in some quarters to a concern with social protection, and in others with participation, community action and development.

The concerns addressed here will seem dated to many people who would describe themselves as socialists because, with the development of new analyses of social conflict, a new kind of socialist politics has also been emerging: a politics concerned not just with egalitarianism but with adjustment of social diversity, and not just with redistribution but with social justice in a broader sense. These issues will be returned to in later chapters.

Part 2

New paradigms: interpretations of a changing society

Chapter 7

Communities and society

Communitarianism

Communitarianism begins from a very different perspective from that of individualism. Individualism shows the world as made of atoms, particles which spin round and never touch each other. Communitarianism begins from the opposite premise: that we are social animals. We are born and grow up in society, not as some theoretical individual but as persons, endowed with a range of relationships, social roles and responsibilities towards other people. According to the communitarian perspective the concept of individualism tends to be treated as something which is abstract, in contrast to the reality of the community. Individualism cannot be treated as a vacuum; the individual can only be understood in the context of others, and the issues of freedom, choice and identity are rooted in social relationships. There is no such thing as the 'unencumbered self'; we all have attachments and it is these attachments which give life meaning. MacIntyre writes that

> we all approach our own circumstances as bearers of a particular social identity. I am someone's son or daughter, someone else's cousin or uncle; I am a citizen of this or that city, a member of this or that guild or profession; I belong to this clan, that tribe, this nation. Hence what is good for me has to be good for one who inhabits these roles.[1]

These roles are social – they define relationships, rights and duties – but they are also distinctive; each person has a different set of roles and that identifies the person's place in society. This is closely identifiable with the organic view of society favoured by some conservatives: 'Man is born into society, into a family and into a nation and, by the mere fact of existence, assumes inescapable duties towards his fellows and is endowed with the rights of membership of that society.'[2]

The implication of these roles is that although people have rights and responsibilities, each person's rights and responsibilities are different. Morality depends on the relative position of each person; what is right for one person may be wrong for another. Universalism, of the kind identified in discussions on 'universal human rights', starts from the assumption that we are all at root the same. Communitarianism begins from a different point, which is the sociological view of the person, and argues that we are all different, and that different rules consequently apply. This position is 'particularist'; it implies that the moral codes which apply to each person are particular to that person's situation, rather than universal.

The argument has been used both from the left and the right of the political spectrum. Left-wing critics have used it to criticise the simplistic assumptions of liberals who seem to assume that everyone lives in isolation from other people. Right-wingers have used it to counter socialist arguments for the imposition of a universal morality on everyone in a society: Charvet's objection to egalitarianism is that inequalities reflect the differential social circumstances associated with different social roles, and the values placed on those roles.[3]

Communitarianism is an attractive and persuasive approach. The premises it begins from are much closer to social reality than individualism; that gives them a strong intellectual appeal. They are also appealing emotionally: communitarianism 'feels' right, because it reflects a system of codes which we hold anyway. For conservatives, it helps to model the social order which they treasure; for socialists, it ties in with the elements of socialist thought which build on the importance of social relationships and collective action.

Then the problems start. Consider an example of which individualists are critical: the issue of female circumcision. From an individualist perspective, female circumcision is abhorrent: it involves imposed suffering, risks to individual health, the loss of pleasure and self-expression for the individual, and the subjection of women. But what, from a communitarian perspective, is wrong with it? If moral codes and responsibilities are defined in a social context, the test which applies is whether the act is meaningful and whether it accords with moral codes. There is nothing in communitarianism which implies that people should be equal – if Charvet is right, the reverse is true – and objections to the domination of women generally rely on a universalist moral code, not on the particular situation. That, of course, is the defence made of the practice by the proponents of female circumcision: this, they say, is part of our culture and our society, and frankly it is none of your business.

Communitarianism equally makes a strong argument for discrimination, in the sense of offering preference to some people over others. The social relationships of family and community imply that people have special responsibilities to the people they are closest to, responsibilities which go over and above the responsibilities they have to others. (An extreme communitarian might not agree that we have any responsibility to the world in general; a moderate version might accept some universal human rights.) But offering special favours to family and close friends can have negative consequences, including the maintenance of privilege and the exclusion of outsiders. Nepotism, literally the appointment of relatives to favoured positions, is generally disapproved of because it leads to people occupying roles in which they are neither qualified or competent, but it is important to recognise why it occurs. People want to do the best for the people they are closest to, and they may feel there is a moral obligation on them to try. The exclusion of outsiders happens because the favours shown to insiders do not leave space for them; if people give preference to their family, then people in richer families will prosper and poor families will not, and if people favour people within their own community, ethnic minorities will suffer. The National Front in France campaigns on the slogan 'French People First'. It is a subtle appeal not simply to racial prejudice, but to moral sentiments which many people share.

Spheres of social action

Liberals have generally taken the view that state intervention is undesirable, and liable to threaten the security of the individual; Hayek's argument, that any extension of state powers was dangerous, was very influential for the New Right. Conservatives have generally favoured state intervention for the purposes of maintaining social order. Communitarian arguments, by contrast, suggest that there are areas – or spheres – in which some intervention may be legitimate, and others might not be. It may be legitimate, for example, to argue that the state should intervene in the economic sphere and not in the family – though the dominant model in much of Europe is Christian Democracy, which tends to favour moral intervention in the family and *laissez-faire* in relation to economics.

The idea of spheres of activity is an old one. The concept of 'sphere sovereignty' was outlined in Chapter 5; the argument was made that different types of activity, like business, arts or the family, reflected the diversity of God's creation and should be considered each as sacrosanct, and subject to different rules from the others. Authority in each sphere developed in relation to the natural order that prevailed within the sphere. Michael Walzer's use of these ideas applies the concept of spheres to a range of social issues. Walzer argues that the concept of social justice is meaningless because it has first to be placed in some kind of social context.

> In a world of particular cultures, competing conceptions of the food, scarce resources, elusive and expansive needs, there isn't going to be a single formula, universally applicable. There isn't going to be a single universally approved path that carries us from a notion like, say, 'fair shares' to a comprehensive list of the goods to which that notion applies. Fair shares of what?[4]

Walzer argues that the standards which apply in relation to spheres like law, commerce or family relations are different. This view is sometimes referred to as 'pluralism', though it is pluralist in a specialised sense of the word; it refers to a plurality of moral codes.

The argument for differentiating spheres has a certain amount to commend it. Like communitarianism, it reflects the moral perceptions which most people actually adopt – very few people, when we come down to it, really think that relations in the family should be run on the same lines as the criminal justice system, or that personal relationships and business should both work on a principle of fair exchange. Unlike communitarianism, it is not intrinsically prejudicial or exclusive; it is possible to make out a case for intervention or group action in specific contexts, according to the sphere which is being discussed. It is controversial, though, for two reasons. One is that if the principle is accepted, then cherished values, like individual liberty, human dignity or respect for persons, cannot be adopted as simple and absolute moral principles; they have to be deconstructed and defended in specific contexts. Second, the spheres have to be defined, and there may be conflicts, and contradictions between them. There is an evident overlap between the spheres of the family, gender and sexuality, but it is very debatable whether the same principles can be held to apply to each.

Social responsibility

What responsibility do people have to other people, or to the society they live in? This is several questions bundled into one. It is a sociological question, concerned with the relationships that people have to each other. It is a moral question, concerned with the relationships which people ought to have to each other. And it is a political question, concerned with the kind of rules by which people, communities and governments should be guided.

The question is problematic only for individualists; any other kind of theory works on the basis that there is some kind of social interaction which has a moral element. The basis of these principles was often religious, and religious believers tend to trace their sense of obligation back to their faith but, equally, the major world religions can be seen to have absorbed many of the dominant social values of earlier times. The central moral concept of a feudal society was the concept of duty; people had duties to God and to others in society, both above them and below them. It was possible to have duties towards people without implying any rights: the duty to give charity and the duty to the poor were duties to God and the social structure, not to the poor themselves. The idea of rights was an innovation, a translation of the principle of duty into something which adhered in the people to whom the duty was owed.

Religious views of society still tend to emphasise duties, rather than rights. Judaism has a structured view of obligation, with the first priority going to one's own community. Maimonides, writing in the twelfth century, suggested eight degrees of benevolence, the highest being to help someone from one's own community to become independent, the second being a gift where neither the donor nor the recipient know each other's identity, and the eighth being gifts given begrudgingly.[5] There was particular concern in this for the dignity of the recipient. Early Christianity emphasised the importance of charity as a duty to God, rather than to the recipient; Lutheranism later reinterpreted the duty as being communal, laying down ordinances for the foundation of a community chest.[6]

The Catholic church emphasises the duty of solidarity, which is 'a firm and persevering determination to commit oneself to the common good, that is . . . the good of all and of each individual, because we are all really responsible for each other'.[7] Solidarity affects both the individual and social groups. Individuals are bound into relationships of solidarity by virtue of their social position, but they can also enter into solidaristic arrangements through consent and mutual aid. This principle, associated with the development of mutualities, was central to the linking of solidarity with the idea of social insurance in the nineteenth century. But solidarity can also refer, in a more general sense, to fraternity – a sense of fellowship or social cohesion – and in recent years the term solidarity has come to stand more for redistribution than for mutualist arrangements.

Catholic social teaching goes further by structuring the sense of obligation expressed in the principle of solidarity through the idea of subsidiarity. Subsidiarity argues that people have the strongest obligations to those they are closest to, and to others who are more distant they have progressively diminishing obligations and a duty to respect this order of things (which implies some limitations on state intervention). Solidaristic relationships are formed through a series of social networks; they change with social relationships, and with one's proximity to the people with whom they are shared. One can imagine, Alfarandi writes, 'a system of concentric circles of solidarity, wider and wider, which goes from the nuclear family to the international community'.[8]

Social exchange theory

Obligations are a part of the social structure; in so far as they are the basis for social roles, status and rights, they could be seen as the foundation of that structure. The fullest account of the development of obligations was made in the 1960s and 1970s in the form of social exchange theory, which argued that the root of many social obligations and patterns of behaviour could be interpreted in terms of a 'norm of reciprocity'.[9] In virtually every society, there is a norm which determines that people feel an obligation to make a return for the things they receive. Balanced exchange takes place when people make direct return for what they receive, and this is fundamental to economic activity. Homans seeks to explain the growth of status in terms of exchange; he suggests that the effect of imbalanced or unequal exchange between individuals is that people receive status in order to redress the balance.[10] Blau extends the analysis to relationships in the wider society.[11] Pinker uses the idea to explain the stigmatisation of the recipients of social welfare: because they are unable to reciprocate, their status is diminished.[12]

There is also, however, generalised exchange, in which people make return, not to a person who has given them things, but to someone else. The model of this kind of exchange came from anthropology: the Kula ring, a ritualised system of exchange in the Trobriand Islands, was the model taken by Marcel Mauss for his analysis of the role of the gift in society.[13] Gifts could be used to create obligations, and even to subdue people – in North America, some tribes exercised 'potlach', a substitute for war which consisted of aggressive giving. We are linked by extended chains of obligations. Parents give to children, not necessarily because the children will make return to them, but because their own parents provided for them. People contribute to voluntary social security, not with the certainty that they will get their contributions back, but on the assurance that the support they give to others will ultimately be extended to them if the occasion demands. This was the basis on which government-based social security systems developed in many countries. Titmuss was to take the principle as the basis for his analysis of the 'gift relationship'; people's actions in giving blood were a paradigm of generalised reciprocity, where giving and receiving were part of a wide circle of interdependence.[14]

Who is my stranger?

The question 'who is my stranger?' was put by Titmuss. By it he meant to ask what our responsibility was to other people in society, who we may have never met and do not know. Intellectually, Titmuss's work on *The Gift Relationship* drew on the insights of social exchange theory.

Titmuss's own response was based largely in the Christian socialism which shaped his own work and ideas. Christianity has traditionally represented the acceptance of obligations to strangers as a sign of particular virtue, with the parable of the Good Samaritan standing as the paradigm for altruistic conduct. But the Good Samaritan is not necessarily a model for the development of social obligation; it is concerned not with obligation, but actions that go beyond obligation, and not with mutual aid, but in the virtue of helping someone who falls outside the circle of social contact within which such charity would ordinarily be exercised.

The main lesson can be taken to be that if one accepts responsibilities to people who are very distant socially, one should accept even more strongly obligations to people who are not so distant. This is the pattern of obligations implied in the Catholic concept of solidarity, discussed earlier. Sahlins suggests that in many ways our social proximity is determined by the pattern of exchange we engage in with others. Among those with whom we are intimate, such as family and close friends, the normal pattern of exchange is generalised. As relationships become more distant, the pattern of exchange is more formally balanced. At the extreme, contact with whom there is the greatest social distance may be 'negative exchange' – a transaction which has the appearance of exchange, but where there may be self-seeking or competitive behaviour, and possibly grudging or negative feelings.[15] This pattern tends to emerge in some forms of business exchange; Sahlins suggests that this may also appear in the donation of resources for the poor, who may be held in low esteem as a result of their dependency but to whom obligations are recognised nevertheless.

Social cohesion

The idea of social cohesion – the persistence of social relationships – is often seen as problematic in sociology: it is particularly difficult for conflict theorists, who have to explain why society does not immediately fall apart. Some of their explanations are based in the study of power as a means for the maintenance of social divisions, and will be returned to in a later chapter.

Solidarity as social cohesion

Solidarity is sometimes seen as a source of cohesion in its own right, and sometimes as a mechanism which can help to reinforce social ties. The Catholic use of the term is not the only way in which it is understood; the term is in widespread use. Durkheim used the term to refer to different types of social organisation, in discussion of the division of labour.[16] 'Mechanical solidarity' occurred in relatively undeveloped societies, in which labour was not specialised and people would attempt to create their own products; the main source of 'social solidarity' lay in relations of obligation and exchange, and the principal social unit would be the family or tribe. 'Organic solidarity' represented the interdependence which occurred in a more developed economy, as the division of labour became more diverse and each person specialised. Under these conditions, Durkheim suggested, a collective consciousness might emerge. This model has never had much direct influence on policy or on later analysis (though there is an argument to be made that Titmuss's 'social division of welfare', one of the seminal influences in the development of social policy, was based in Durkheim's ideas[17]). For practical purposes, the importance of the idea is the belief that social cohesion is promoted through involvement in economic activity and the division of labour. The Single European Act contains a general aim of promoting 'economic and social cohesion', and there is a protocol to the Maastricht Treaty concerned with the subject.

Functionalism

One of the most controversial forms of analysis of social structures is the attribution of 'functions' to different elements or processes. Ascribing a function to an object says that the object is used by someone for a purpose. Cars, for example, are used to travel, to transport goods, to make statements about status, and to make profits for the motor industry. They do other things – like running people over and polluting the atmosphere – but these are not functions, because they are not done for a purpose. Functionalism is the attribution of functions to different aspects of social structure.

The controversy over functionalism stems from two quite unrelated arguments. The first is based in a simple mistake, but we have to get it out of the way before considering the real arguments. This is the view that functionalists are conservatives who believe that every social rule is useful and serves a desirable purpose. Some conservatives have been functionalist: Edmund Burke argued that social rules were generally there because they had been tried and found to be good and useful, and that we should be very wary about changing them on that account. But many conservatives are not functionalists, and many functionalists are not conservative. Most of the people who make functionalist arguments nowadays are neo-Marxists, like Offe (who argues that the welfare state helps to legitimate the capitalist system).[18] Marxist analysis is strongly functionalist in this sense: social disadvantage, the class structure, and the policies which states pursue are widely seen as functional for the capitalist system.

The second, and much more important, argument concerns whether or not social phenomena can be said to have any purpose. This suggests that someone wants what happens to happen, and that some process exists by which it can be brought about. Marxists attribute the process to the exercise of power and the operation of the economic system. The American functionalists, like Parsons and Merton, argued that social structures served functions in a rather broader sense; certain forces served to hold society together simply in the sense that society would cease to exist without them.[19] Lévi-Strauss, an anthropologist who has been described as a 'structural functionalist', argued that the taboo on incest is functional in this sense. Lévi-Strauss's argument, in a nutshell, is that a society in which incest is permitted will find that people do not marry outside their own families, with the result that there is reduced social contact and a failure to form and build the social relationships which intermarriage develops.[20] Functionalism offers, then, an explanation of how society coheres, and the mechanisms by which norms and morals which promote cohesion are maintained. The main critique of this position comes from individualists, who argue that because social action has to be understood as an aggregate of individual analysis the idea that there are social purposes is meaningless; from those who argue that it is overly deterministic; and from those who see the process of cohesion as the result of the exercise of power or the dominant interests of particular groups in society.

Parsons and system integration

The problem of social order was the central issue addressed by Talcott Parsons, who was also the leading functionalist. Parsons described four processes which worked to ensure cohesion. These were adaptation, because the ability to adjust to change and to the environment is essential for social order; goal attainment, where people and social groups try to do the things they want to do; pattern maintenance, through the values, beliefs and culture which people are socialised into; and integration, which refers to the way in which the social system balances the concerns of different, and possibly conflicting, elements. Different aspects of society emphasise different principles – the political process, for example, tends to emphasise goal attainment, while the legal process tends to emphasise integration – but there are elements of each process in every aspect of society.[21]

It is difficult to think of a writer who has been more thoroughly traduced in the literature; Parsons is widely represented as an arch-conservative with no understanding of social conflict. Parsons may have been a conservative – certainly, when Marxism became anathema in the USA, Parsons traded on his conservative and anti-Marxist reputation to defend Marxist sociologists from attack – but he also took strong positions against racism and fascism, and in terms of US politics he might reasonably be considered a radical. Haralambos, in fairness summarising the literature rather than levelling these charges himself, writes that Parsons assumes that there is consensus in society; that he fails to consider the situation in which some people dominate others; and (citing Lockwood) that 'in focusing on the contributing of norms and values to social order, Parsons largely fails to recognize the conflicts of interest which tend to produce instability and disorder.'[22] This is all rubbish, which it has largely been possible to maintain simply because Parsons' writing is so pompous and turgid that hardly anyone nowadays can be bothered to read it. Parsons was not by any means blind to social conflict or division; on the contrary, Lee and Newby argue, 'whatever else might be unsatisfactory in the theory, it is built upon the idea that society presupposes competing, even irreconcilable, elements and that constant changes and adjustments have to be made as a result.'[23]

Parsons looked in detail at cases in which order seem to be maintained despite very fundamental conflicts, and on that basis he made special studies of Nazi Germany and the position of African Americans in the USA,[24] which in view of the conflicts they generated needed explanation as to why they did not lead to social collapse.

From the point of view of social policy rather than sociology, the importance of Parsons' work is twofold. First, Parsons was concerned to show the mechanisms by which different and contradictory elements in society could create the appearance of social order; the issues he identified, including the application of culture, the adaptation of the organism to the social environment and the constant shifting of social norms, are all key issues in the relationship of sociology to social policy. Although the language which Parsons used is not widely referred to, the concepts are, and

Parsons's agenda directed sociologists to consider issues, like health care[25] and race,[26] which had previously been considered as of marginal importance in sociology. Second, Parsons employed a series of methods which were profoundly influential in social science, and which are still used in the analysis of sociology and social policy. These included the application of systems theory to the analysis of society, the tabulation of different principles in order to examine their interactions, and testing the general theory against complex and difficult counter-examples.

Social policy and social cohesion

Though it is not the sense in which the term is principally used, social policy is sometimes represented as a policy for society. As such, social policy plays an important role in the maintenance of social order. From the point of view of Marxists, social policy has the functional roles of reproducing society and servicing the forces of accumulation. A conservative view might see social policy as a means for maintaining social order. This element is visible in the emphasis on social cohesion in the European Union. Social cohesion is taken to refer to the integrity of the social fabric,[27] and the problem of exclusion – exclusion, specifically, from solidaristic social relationships – 'threatens the social cohesion of each Member State and of the Union as a whole.'[28] Such poverty is threatening the cohesion of the Union, and there are 'cracks appearing in the social fabric'.[29] The rhetoric seems overblown; the fear of the poor as a kind of alien horde which threatens to engulf respectable society has been a recurring theme in writing about poverty for over 200 years, but it is hard to sustain. In the chapters which follow, though, we will consider some of the issues of social change and social division which are at the root of this perception.

Chapter 8

New views of the economy

Economic processes: production

Although the economic system of the world is often referred to as 'capitalist', there is a considerable gap between the theory of capitalism and economic production in practice. The dominant view of the economy, on both right and left, is that the economy works by a set of mechanisms. Goods are produced in order to be exchanged, the principal medium of exchange is monetary, and in consequence the production of goods is related directly to financial conditions. The production of goods for exchange is identifiable in terms of the pursuit of profit, which provides the motivation for economic action.

This received wisdom is, at best, a half-truth. There are three main problems. The first is that, even within the confines of the conventional model, the economy is complex, and does not actually work on a common set of principles at all. The characterisation of production as being held in private hands is an over-simplification; different operators have different motivations and modes of activity. Even within a conventional view of the economy, capitalists (people who own and control the means of production) nestle cheek by jowl with feudal aristocrats, corner grocers, and multinational corporate structures. The production of an individual operator (like, say, the work of an independent medical practitioner) is governed by different criteria from those of a medium-sized firm, and differently again from those of a corporate enterprise.

The second problem is that, within a modern economy, there are many other motivations for action besides the profit motive. The public sector often works to different criteria from those of the private sector. Within the private sector, there are further sub-divisions. For one thing, the ownership of economic enterprises is often separated from their management, with the effect that the profit motive may be subordinated to other criteria, like long-term growth, security or career development. For another, there is in many countries an identifiable group of industries which work explicitly on a non-profit basis. This is most strikingly the case in the financial sector, where mutualities have played an important part in pensions, insurance and housing provision, though it also applies in sectors like medicine and education.

The third reservation is that substantial parts of the productive process are removed from the world in which commodities are traded and exchanged. Examples are social relationships, domestic labour, parenting, and large parts of leisure activities – in other words, a great deal of what really matters in life. As specialists in welfare, we are concerned mainly with how people live their lives, and involvement in the economy is only part of that.

The behaviour of the firm

In formal economics, the assumption is generally made that firms exist to make profits, and that they intend to maximise their profits – that is, make as much profit as they possibly can. But making as much money as possible is not necessarily the best strategy to undertake: trying to milk consumers in the short term will lead to losses in the long term; confining production to what is most efficient may leave the market open to other suppliers; and making too much money invites the attention of competitors (or worse, vampires who, unlike their fictional counterparts, fly around economic markets in broad daylight). There is a theory of the firm quite distinct from the formal predictions of economic analysis, which tries to model what firms will do with a range of objectives – maximising profits over the long term rather than the short term, maximising growth. The most common pattern is a form of compromise, often referred to as 'satisficing' – a combination of satisfaction and maximisation.

In *The New Industrial State*, Galbraith outlined a new explanation of the behaviour and motivation of the modern industrial firm.[1] Galbraith was interested not in the activities of the local plumber or shop-owner, people who own and control their firms, but with the large, conglomerate firms which have come to dominate international markets. The basic propositions of his argument are as follows.

1 From the perspective of the modern industrial firm, capital – the finance for production – is abundant. The commodity which is most often in scarce supply is expertise.

2 The more advanced the technology which is being applied, the more difficult it is for any one person to have command over it all. The characteristic method of production is teamwork, in which a range of specialists each contribute their expertise to the development of a product. There is a strong division of labour between the specialists.

3 Firms have to be structured in a form which allows each specialist to exercise control in the area of their speciality. This precludes simple hierarchies, in which people are told what to do by the person immediately above them. The structure is, rather, corporate and collegiate.

4 The firms are run by these teams, and that means that they are run in their interests. This leads to a different kind of motivation from a concern with profits (which mainly benefit shareholders and owners). Their priorities are likely to be high salaries, perks (extra benefits from employment) and secure employment.

5 Corporate, high-technology firms have a vested interest in ensuring that their production remains corporate and high-tech. This is what guarantees the security of the corporate team. They are concerned to exclude competitors, avoid devaluation of the technology through the development of lower-technology alternatives (which would mean that their position as guardians of that technology would also be devalued) and promote the advantages of their approach. This leads corporate industries consistently to promote advanced applications of their technology – cars rather than bicycles, whole-body scanners rather than preventive medicine, industrialised building rather than traditional methods of house construction.

Galbraith's models are firms engaged in defence and car production, but the arguments apply to any complex, high-technology production – including, for example, information technology, house construction and health care.

Galbraith's model is a strikingly convincing and accurate portrayal of a particular part of the industrial process, and of the behaviour of some firms within it. But how appropriate is it as a general analysis? There are three reservations to make. The first is that there are so many different kinds of firm engaged in economic activity, including not only production but also finance and distribution, that generalisations do not clearly hold up. Second, an analysis which interprets behaviour in terms of structural factors is only telling part of the story. Ideas about management are formed from a variety of sources, and some of them – like efficiency, Total Quality Management, or the learning organisation – are rooted not so much in the experience of particular types of structure as in an ideology of how firms ought to be managed. It is interesting to note that the current theory of management dominant in health care is a simple, hierarchical one, in which a 'manager' is put in charge of everything and everyone. This model is drawn from the way that supermarkets are run, not high-technology firms, and it does not fit the circumstances – but wherever possible, the circumstances are being made to fit.

Fordism and post-Fordism

One particularly influential view of the productive process has been the description of production as 'post-Fordist'. Fordism was a method of mass production, based on a strict division of labour exemplified by the assembly line in Henry Ford's car plants. It is closely associated with the model of 'scientific management' developed by Frederick Taylor, also known as 'Taylorism', which was based on the breakdown of industrial activity into definable tasks. This approach has often been criticised for the deskilling, and dehumanizing, of labour. Although both Fordism and Taylorism were widely practised, neither could be said substantially to have dominated the processes of industrial production; they were important in particular industries (such as food production and car manufacturing). There are generally recognised problems of rigidity in production – the system, once established, can be difficult to change – and alienation of the labour force.

Jessop describes four aspects of Fordism. It was a pattern of production, and a labour process – a method of using labour for mass production. It was a model for economic growth (associated with Keynesianism), describing a system of mass production in a high-consumption economy. It was a means of regulating the economy, involving large-scale, centralised, managed corporations. And it described a pattern of society – the paradigm of 'modernity', which is discussed later in this book.[2] The importance of Fordism for welfare was the establishment of stable, often relatively high-paid employment for large numbers of people – a pattern of employment which is at the core of particular models of social protection (particularly the Bismarckian systems of central Europe, in which benefits are conditional on work record).

Fordism, however, was always limited in its scope, and a number of writers have argued that it has given way to 'post-Fordism'. Post-Fordism represents a new pattern of work, based on a flexible division of labour. Like Fordism, the idea extends beyond issues in the structure of production: 'If "post-Fordism" exists', Hall writes, 'it is as much a description of cultural as of economic change.'[3] Post-Fordist production is small scale, and based on collaborative group activity. This flexibility makes it possible to adapt products to a changing market, but it also has the disadvantage for employees that their tenure in employment is very limited. For workers with limited skills, this can imply precarious employment and marginalisation. This, in turn, has posed challenges for welfare states which have depended either on full employment or on the work record of the employee as the key to gain access to social protection.[4] If the welfare state does not adapt to this change, Sabel suggests, the welfare state would still survive, but it 'would look like a more ramshackle version of its current self.'[5]

The labour market

The conventional liberal view of the labour market is built around the idea of a competition for labour, in which lots of people wish to employ workers, and lots of people wish to work. But the emphasis on expertise in corporate production has distorted this market; there may be many people who want to work, but they do not necessarily have the specific skills or experience which the prospective employer is looking for. There can be, then, several markets rather than one. The central argument falls between macro-economists – economists who look at the whole economy – and micro- or labour market economists. There are market economists who are interested in the macro-economics of labour markets, who seek to provide links between macro levels of unemployment and wages levels, in contrast to market economists who tend to look at micro labour markets, unemployment and wages.

Macro-economists seek to emphasise the context of general labour markets, while micro-economists aim to explain how rational agents in the context of disaggregated labour markets produce different responses to changes in the levels of unemployment and wages. According to the micro-economists some workers, because of their skills and knowledge differences, are located in sectors which are less vulnerable to competitive markets, at least in the short term. This applies equally to public sector workers, including teachers or doctors who do not sell a product directly to the public.

In dealing with the problem of unemployment therefore, macro- and micro-economists tend to look at different variables. Micro-economists are concerned with the strategies available to different workers in aiming to influence the labour market. Micro-economists therefore tend to emphasise the process of disaggregated labour markets. Macro-economists are interested in the process of wage determination, of explaining other macro variables including the rate of inflation, interest rates and changes in the currency. These are likely to influence wage demands and therefore the rate of unemployment.

Insiders and outsiders

Changes in the pattern of industrial production imply changes in the nature of employment. Some economists have identified workers as 'insiders' or 'outsiders'. The insider/outsider group interpretation suggested that workers are either 'core' workers and in employment or they are at the periphery of the labour market. Core workers tend to be at the heart of the firm: workers who have specialist skills and knowledge on which the organisation depends. The core group tends to have easier access to management decisions. Managers are aware of the cost of losing key workers, the cost of replacement in terms of time and investment in skills. Core workers offer stability and continuation of production and firms are aware that the demand for core workers is high so that poaching through higher wage incentives by other firms can make certain firms vulnerable and at risk. Core workers will therefore enter bargains with their employers which ensure their retention, so that even during periods of economic slowdown when demand falls, employers are likely to 'hoard' these core workers as they await an economic upturn.

In contrast, workers on the periphery of the organisation tend to be treated as the outsiders compared to the core workers. Outsiders continue to stay on the outside of the organisation. Firms do not attempt to invest in the human capital of workers who are at the margin of the organisation or attempt to integrate them into the organisation. Outsiders are seen as easily replaced or made redundant during economic slowdown. There is no attempt to hoard periphery workers, because they can be easily replaced and retrained at short notice in an economic upturn. The wages of the outsider group reflects their outsider status, namely that if they do not like their rates of pay they can easily look elsewhere as employers can always find new workers to replace them.

The insider/outsider theory questions the assumption held by market economists that there is a link between those in work and those out of work, namely that those out of work can influence wage levels by under-bidding the price of those who are employed. The reason why the insiders (the employed people) are not directly threatened by the outsiders (the unemployed) is because of the cost incurred by employers in accepting the process of under-bidding by outsiders. Firms are likely to lose on their productivity if they are involved in high labour turnover. Irrespective of the skills of the labour force, the insiders always have more knowledge of the productive process than the outsiders. High labour turnover is associated with low labour morale and adversely effects productivity.

The dual labour market

The idea of a 'dual labour market' is another way of representing the fracture which has appeared in the nature of employment. There is not a single working population; labour supply cannot be treated as a homogeneous factor. Labour markets are segmented by class, gender and race. These markets are often tightly segregated with little cross-influence between these labour markets. Male white workers tend to be insulated in highly skilled occupations. There is a core of male white workers who are highly skilled, or have access to specialist knowledge, who belong to trade unions and professional associations and who seek to protect their income differentials from other workers through pre-entry closed shops and other exclusive strategies. Workers who enjoy access to specialist skills may seek, as rational agents, to combine together to protect their skills and also to exclude others with barriers to entry into these skills. Engineering workers, for example, set specific durations for apprenticeships before new workers can be classified as qualified engineers. Barristers have ensured that their profession is kept separate from solicitors as do consultants from doctors in health care. This form of segregation results in income differentials between groups of workers who feel they have skills and knowledge to sell in the market where supply is restricted.

By contrast, male workers from ethnic minorities tend to have more access to manual occupations which require little training, occupations which tend to be low paid and highly seasonal. Ethnic minority workers tend to be more vulnerable to the experience of unemployment than their majority counterparts. There is no direct competition between minority and majority workers.

There are segmented labour markets for women also; women tend to enter occupations which are part time and low paid, but they also tend to have more access to professional occupations in the public sector including the teaching and the medical professions than do black women workers, who tend to be confined to a more narrow labour market which is part-time, low-paid employment. Women from ethnic minorities have less access to professional occupations in the public sector than other women.

One of the implications of this change in the labour market is that there are those who will be marginalised within it. Their work is of low status and earning power; when work is scarce, they are particularly vulnerable to unemployment. In France, these kinds of conditions are generally referred to in terms of 'précarité'; Matza and Miller describe the situation in terms of 'sub-employment'.[6]

Consumption

The analysis of the economy is often concerned with the process of production – how things are made, and on what terms. The issue of how things are consumed is no less important, and here the traditional models give much less guidance. The conventional representation of consumption in economic theory shows the consumer as an individual, who makes rational choices between alternatives. The argument is not that people are all rational but, that if people's behaviour is taken in aggregate, the general trend of behaviour will follow predictable patterns. People in aggregate attempt to increase their welfare by increasing their use of material goods; to make the best use of their resources, they prefer when other things are equal to pay less for the same item; they will choose what they want rather than what they do not want.

There are examples which contradict any of these basic propositions. People in aggregate do not always want more goods: there
is a problem when the increasing number of goods, like the
number of motor cars, starts to detract from aggregate welfare,
and some consumer movements (especially 'green' and conservation
activity) consist of privileged groups trying to prevent others from
expanding their activities. People do not always want to pay less:
there are status goods, like housing, which are worth more simply
because people want to pay more for them. People do not always
choose what they want, because they do not necessarily have control
over their choices; when old people go into residential care, the decision tends to be made for them by a professional or a family
member. These are important exceptions, and they have specific
implications for the fields in which they occur, but they do not disprove the basic propositions; they only qualify them, implying that
there are grounds for caution about applying them too widely. The
analysis of housing markets is bedeviled by puzzled economists who
are convinced that their principles ought to apply, and they would if
only the market was able to operate properly.[7] They wouldn't.

This leads to a second pattern of analysis, which represents consumption in terms of interest groups. There are identifiable groups
in relation to particular markets. This can be interpreted in a pluralistic, diverse sense: there are 'green' consumers, female consumers,
home owners, young people, and so forth. The categories are diverse
and complex, with considerable potential for overlap. The differentiation of consumer groups implies that there are different markets
for different kinds of commodity, not simply in the sense that
people do not go shopping for cars and health care at the same
time, but that the markets in these commodities work in different
ways. A former director of Kentucky Fried Chicken, working as
the manager of a private health firm in the UK, is credited with
the comment that there is no difference in principle in selling
health care and Kentucky Fried Chicken. To many analysts of
social policy, that statement seems, at the very least, implausible.
The consumers of health care often have specific requirements
for treatment in which substitutability of alternatives is limited; in
consequence, they have limited choice and highly inelastic
demand. They also have restricted knowledge of potential courses
of action, and considerable constraints on their range of action,
both monetary and non-monetary.

The third representation is the view that there are consumption classes (and in some cases, consumption 'cleavages' where class interests lead to radically different patterns of behaviour). Consumption is stratified according to economic and social circumstances, and the patterns of consumption reflect other patterns of social stratification. Rex and Moore applied this analysis to housing studies with a concept of 'housing class'.[8] (This use of the idea of 'class' is identified with Weber, who sees class in terms of a common economic position; it contrasts with the Marxian use of the term, which defines class in relation to the means of production.) In Rex and Moore's analysis, different patterns of housing tenure reflected important differences in the economic position of different groups of people. Housing was important enough, in turn, to affect other aspects of people's lives – including their pattern of consumption, and their social status. These factors interacted to identify a specific class, based on their consumption of housing.

The importance of consumption is recognised in the concept of 'dual politics'. This idea was developed by Marxists who recognised that the patterns of consumption in a society did not comfortably fit the Marxist model. Production appeared, to Marxists, to be stratified, serving the interests of a ruling class who owned and controlled the means of production. The corporatist model revised was consistent with that, because it explained how control could be exercised through a complex economy. Consumption, by contrast, was pluralistic and diverse; the politics of consumption has to be understood, not in terms of class, but of factions and interest groups.[9]

Dual politics was developed essentially as a modification of Marxist arguments, an attempt to fuse different patterns of analysis. The most obvious flaw in this rests in the analysis of production; it relies on an acceptance of Marxist premises, which fit the circumstances uncomfortably. Conversely, the analysis of consumption depends on a view that consumption patterns are not structured hierarchically, which is difficult to reconcile with analyses of gender and race. The main appeal of the model lies in the recognition that there is no reason why production and consumption have to be analysed in the same terms. Production may be structured and patterned, while consumption is pluralistic and diffuse; the converse may be true. The important insight is that they do not have to be explained in the same way, and on the same terms.

The operation of the market

The analysis of markets lies at the core of much of what is done in economics, and the arguments are familiar ones. Under certain assumptions, the operation of a free market has been argued to lead to an efficient allocation of resources. Production and consumption are brought into balance, or 'equilibrium'. There have to be multiple producers competing with each other: competition forces producers to keep their prices low, but prices which are too low will drive people out of business. There have to be multiple purchasers, who are free to choose whether or not to buy the commodities which are being sold. When there is a shortage of goods, people demand more, and the price rises, encouraging producers into the market. When there is a surplus, prices fall and production is discouraged. This process is automatic, the 'hidden hand' favoured by market liberals.

The problems of this theory should be familiar. Even within the constraints of the theory, there is a problem of market failure – that particular conditions may apply which mean that the market does not allocate resources efficiently. The first set of problems relates to the social implications of the private market. There is, for example, the problem of externalities. The right of the individual to self-interest might incur costs to others, and the probability that individual self-interest might therefore not result in economic efficiency. One example is the condition of the environment: the need to protect the environment is a communal one, based in the concern for the ecology and the earth's life cycle; such a problem cannot be left to individual self-interest. Another is investment in human capital. The concept of self-interest addresses issues of education as a form of investment in the person; that is when education becomes a decision of investment in human capital. Individuals making decisions about their personal investment costs will put a higher cost on investment than a government does for society. If a higher investment in human capital is proved to be highly correlated with higher living standards for the whole community – thus affording better health care, more care for the elderly and a better environment – then that society would see investment in the individual human capital as an investment in the community also.

A second problem is the issue of public goods. The logic of market economics would suggest that all activities have the property of being commodities for which there are likely to be suppliers and consumers. But there are certain public goods which do not easily transfer into commodities and prices. Examples of public goods would include the provision of parks, roads, street lighting, sewers, policing and defence. The benefits derived cannot simply be identified as costs to identifiable individuals.

The private market also has inefficiencies in its operation. There may be economics of scale and efficiency in a publicly provided service, like a national health service. There are commodities, like social services for the vulnerable, in which choice is difficult to exercise, and the market has to rely on alternative mechanisms (notably insurance). And there are problems in coverage, both because some people are unable to demand services effectively, and because the efficient delivery of services requires producers to select between options – offering those aspects of services which can be done at the lowest unit cost, and excluding those services which cannot.

The positions which are outlined above raise further questions about the operation of the market. Producers are not necessarily profit-maximising; indeed, some forms of production are dominated by corporate management, whose interests may be different. The divisions apparent in the operation of the labour market will not prevent the emergence of multiple consumers, but they do imply for some a degree of economic marginality or exclusion. The implication of consumption cleavages is that demand may be generated by only a section of the population, and that the needs and aspirations of others are discounted.

Economic processes and welfare

For many commentators, there is no real distinction to draw between arguments about economics and arguments about welfare. Economists tend to view welfare in terms of utility, the preferences expressed in the market; 'welfare economics' is concerned with the identification of utilities and the study of how welfare can be maximised. In the field of social policy, Cahill has made a case for extending the subject's field of vision to issues like leisure, transport and shopping, issues which are intimately bound up with the process of production and consumption.[10]

Social policy also has a narrower, more specific focus, however: it began from the study of the social services, and even in its wider sense it is concerned with the application of knowledge about social science to practical issues and problems, with a particular focus on deprivation and disadvantage. The main question for students of social policy is not, then, how these processes affect people in general, but how they affect those who are disadvantaged or excluded. The immediate implications of segmented labour markets are felt most directly in the workplace itself. The impermanence of employment, and the vulnerability of lower paid workers, implies weakness in organised labour, and problems of regulating the market. Issues like health and safety at work, minimum wage regulation or the payment of contributions by employers become difficult to enforce.

Welfare systems have commonly been based on the occupational status of workers within the labour market. The Bismarckian schemes applied in continental Europe based social protection, including health as well as social security, on the industry that a person worked in and on the contribution record of the individual worker. The Beveridge scheme in the UK accepted the possibility of casual or intermittent employment, but still relied on full and stable employment for its financial viability. The implications of flexible and segmented labour markets for this kind of provision are considerable. Without a foundation in stable employment, social insurance becomes the preserve of the relatively privileged – like the system which protects public service workers in southern Europe.[11]

Employment is, then, crucial to the status of disadvantaged people. Marxism traditionally saw the divide as falling between those who worked and those who exploited labour power. The analysis above suggests a more complex picture. There are those who work in secure occupations with a guarantee of social protection; those who work in insecure or precarious occupations, with limited coverage and protection; and those who are economically excluded and unable to participate in the formal economy at all. The failure of the economic system to incorporate people into the processes of production and consumption is a fundamental issue for the study of social policy. Economic mechanisms have to be adapted to provide both for those who are marginal, and for the excluded.

Chapter 9

The global economy

Economic development and growth

Economic development depends crucially on the integration of people into formal economic processes. Involvement in the formal economy does not mean that people are involved in a specific kind of activity, nor that they are involved in a particular pattern of production. What makes the economy 'formal' is that people are involved in a pattern of exchange – whatever they do is exchanged for money, and the money can in turn be exchanged for goods. This may seem obvious, because it is so much taken for granted in the developed economies. In under-developed countries, however, many people are not part of the formal economy. They scratch out a living from the land; they build their own houses from materials they find; they manage with what they can. The movement to a formal economy means that people move out of independent subsistence living into interdependence.

There is a strand of green thinking which argues that economic development is undesirable, and that we are no better off than when humans scratched an existence in the dirt.

> Third World people . . . can control how they feel . . . You go to Sri Lanka and you see the kids happy, happy, happy. You go to America and they're not happy as a race . . . You can be happy living in cardboard boxes.
>
> [People] must not view poverty as a drudge but as a gift. Some of the best things in life are learned when you are poor.[1]

These people may not care whether children die, whether people are crippled by avoidable disease or have to spend their day humping water home, but some of us do. Life is getting better, and economic development is the central reason why this is happening. Economic development produces material goods, offering a range of facilities and in particular substituting soft labour for hard labour. It fosters social integration and interdependency; after the initial problems of industrialisation, which often exacerbate inequality and make people vulnerable, developed societies have had an excellent record of promoting exchange and autonomous action. And it generally produces beneficial side-effects: the last thirty years have seen a spectacular improvement in welfare, with a major reduction in infant mortality, increased longevity, the eradication of major world diseases (notably smallpox) and progressive increases in the number of people who have access to basic amenities, including drinking water and a source of fuel.

The benefits of industrial development are felt not only by the people most immediately involved in the economic process, but by the people they are directly in contact with – families and communities. There is a 'multiplier' effect, sometimes referred to as a 'trickle-down' effect. This term needs clarification, because it has been misused in political arguments, most notably by the Reagan administration in the USA in the 1980s. In the literature on developing countries, it refers to the benefits to the poor of a country's integration into economic processes. 'Trickle-down economic growth . . . has played an important role in reducing poverty when the poor have taken advantage of the trickle coming their way.'[2] In relation to the developed world, it has been used to suggest that poor people are generally better off in a society where more wealth is produced. A rising tide, the cliché goes, lifts all boats. That is much more debatable: the effect of inegalitarian economic growth can be to exclude the poor altogether. Mishra comments: 'a rising economic tide not only does not lift all boats, it can upturn, destroy and sink many boats.'[3]

The process of economic development has its risks and dangers. People become vulnerable in the formal economy in a way which is not true when they are poor.

> Diversified subsistence farmers may be poor but are not vulnerable. When they enter the market by selling specialised cash crops, or raising their earnings by incurring debts, or investing in risky ventures, their incomes rise, but they become

vulnerable. There are trade-offs between poverty and vulner-ability (or between security and income).[4]

In more developed societies there may be polarisation, in which economic benefits and security are confined to a privileged core while others are excluded. Ferrera argues it applies to the developed economies of Southern Europe.[5]

Growth is essential to welfare, for three interrelated reasons. The first is that economic resources are needed to cope both with population increases and the poverty of many people, in the developed world as well as in developing countries. Second, as Anthony Crosland argued, redistribution is only politically possible in conditions of growth. People in the developed world will never accept a reduction of two-thirds of their living standards to support the Third World, any more than people who have high earnings within developed countries would accept major redistribution to the poorest in those countries. In a growing economy, by contrast, it is possible to improve everyone's living standards, and to improve those of the poorest, both relatively and absolutely, by slowing the rate of improvement of the better-off. Third, the formal economy brings people directly into the networks of exchange relationships and reciprocity on which welfare depends. Poverty is not seen only as a question of material resources; it is also linked to people's entitlements,[6] and to their ability to participate in society.[7] In the context of development studies, that depends in practice on inclusion in a formal economy.

Globalisation

The progressive inclusion of less developed economies into formal processes of exchange is at the core of the phenomenon of 'globalisation'. Globalisation refers to the development of a world economy – an economy in which boundaries of nationality and geography are progressively being overcome. The International Monetary Fund (IMF) report on the world economic outlook for 1997 defines globalisation as:

> The growing economic interdependence of countries worldwide through the volume of cross-border transactions in goods and services and of international capital flows, and through the more rapid and widespread diffusion of technology.[8]

According to the IMF definition, globalisation implies the shift towards a more internationalised economy brought about by an increase in trade between countries, an increase in capital inflows and the impact of technology in standardising manufacturing output. International organisations such as the World Bank, GATT (General Agreement on Tariffs and Trade, now the World Trade Organisation) and the European Union have all contributed to liberalisation and competitive markets.

There is a sense, of course, in which there has always been a world economy; international trade, conquest, colonialisation, migration and cultural diffusion are long-established historical patterns. Marx wrote in *The Communist Manifesto*:

> The need of a constantly expanding market for its products chases the bourgeoisie over the whole surface of the globe. It must nestle everywhere, settle everywhere, establish connections everywhere . . . it creates a world after its own image.[9]

What is new is speed, which has led to what David Harvey calls 'time–space compression'.[10] Travel and communications systems have made it possible for firms and financiers to choose location without a serious cost in time. There is rapid movement of capital, goods, services and people. Sociologists have suggested that the growing homogeneity of the economy is reflected in the homogeneity of different societies: with economic interdependence, and a shared foundation of material goods, comes a common currency of culture, ideology and leisure pursuits.

The globalised economy is increasingly linked with the concept of competitiveness and the ability of national economies to retain their share of trade. The globalised economy suggests both an expansion of trade and also an increase in the number of nations involved in trade. The ability of a national economy to 'compete' with other economies is usually discussed within the 'ability to sell approach' and locational attractiveness. The ability to sell approach tends to focus on issues which include relative costs, productivity and exchange rates. By contrast, locational attractiveness is related to the ability to attract foreign direct investment.

The nation-state within the context of the globalised economy is perceived to have no impact on macro-economic policy and attempts to deal with the impact of globalised markets. The failure of the European Exchange Rate Mechanism in the 1990s to deal with the problems of currency speculation and turbulence confirms the limitations, not only of the nation-state, but also of supra-national agreements to deal with a globalised currency market.

The globalised economy could however be seen as an excuse for doing nothing. In a globalised world system, the nation abandons responsibility for major areas of policy such as social or employment policy, but retains responsibility for law and order, and territorial jurisdiction as a means of controlling migration of labour between state boundaries. According to Hirst and Thompson, the concept of globalisation is a godsend for both left and right political thinkers.[11] For the right, globalisation confirms the need to create competitive labour markets, deregulation, more privatisation, reducing the role of government and reducing taxation. By contrast, globalisation confirms to the left the weakness of government and the limitations of reformist and revisionist policy.

Hirst and Thompson's argument is that in the period between 1890 and 1914 the world economy went through a phase of inter-nationalisation and liberalisation of trade. The present process can be explained in terms of a new phase of internationalisation rather than globalisation. The world economy is not globalised while 80 per cent of trade is still located within the top five industrial economies (the European Union is treated as an economic unit), and 80 per cent of foreign direct investment is still within the limits of the advanced industrial economies.

However, whether the world economy is becoming 'globalised' or 'internationalised' it would seem that national economies in the 1990s are now more open to trade, to capital and to the impact of technological change. These factors are increasingly leading to nation-states joining into trade blocs such as the EU or the North American Free Trade Association (NAFTA). These blocs seek to reach agreement around issues of liberalisation and free trade; hence the continuing dispute between the USA, Europe and Japan around issues of subsiding agriculture and airlines. Nation-states are therefore increasingly pooling their national sovereignty in a process of seeking membership of wider trade blocs that would guarantee economic and political stability.

The global economy and deindustrialisation

Globalisation depends on trade, and the logic of exchange demands a degree of specialisation. Countries which engage in trade will be able to identify the areas of production in which they have a 'comparative advantage', and the division of labour which results leads to improvement in the total production which is possible within the world economy.

The process of specialisation has important consequences, however. It means that existing firms which work in the wrong kind of enterprise – like much agriculture in Southern Europe, heavy engineering in Northern Europe or textiles in much of the developed world – will find themselves undercut by producers in other countries. Conversely, specific countries find they have an advantage in particular forms of production – the USA in computer technology, the UK in finance, Japan in electronics – and are able to develop in those industries. The establishment of free trade areas – notably the areas in North America and the European Union – has the important consequence of encouraging this process. This is why the European Community could not simply be a trading area, without some form of protection from the consequences of free trade; the regional funds are intended to compensate specific areas for the problems of dislocation, while the social funds offer support for people who are displaced and for the costs of retraining.

What this has meant, for much of Europe, is a major reduction in manufacturing employment and, in consequence, of industry requiring mass labour. Employment for the group of industrial countries has declined from 28 per cent of the labour force to 18 per cent in 1996. There have been some major differences between countries: the USA experienced the sharpest decline, from 28 per cent in 1965 to 16 per cent in 1994, in contrast to Japan where manufacturing employment during the same period declined more slowly, from 27.4 per cent to 23 per cent in 1994. In the UK, manufacturing total output between 1973 and 1992 increased by 1.3 per cent in contrast with 68 per cent in Japan, 68 per cent in Italy and 55 per cent in the USA. Meanwhile, productivity growth in the UK has grown 78 per cent between 1979 and 1995, and the UK has closed the gap with Germany from 40 per cent to 17 per cent. However, UK jobs in manufacturing between 1964 and 1989 declined by a third against 10 per cent in France and 13 per cent in Germany.

Throughout Northern Europe, the decline in manufacturing has been associated with the concept of deindustrialisation as coalfields, steel plants and textile mills have shut down. Industrial communities have disappeared since the mid-1980s as male workers lost their main source of employment and income. The labour shake-out in manufacturing affected mainly semi-skilled male workers whose jobs were replaced by new technologies. Despite attempts to regenerate these economies, jobs lost in manufacturing have been difficult to replace. The expansion of the service sector has by contrast tended to offer employment which is more part time and low paid and directed mainly at women workers. Long-term male unemployment is a major problem for all the advanced industrial economies.

The break-up of industrial communities had major implications for social policy both in terms of costs to infrastructure but also in the sense that governments have had to fund the labour shake-out through higher unemployment and social security payments. The break-up of communities has resulted in schools having to close down as families moved to seek their employment fortunes elsewhere. Those left behind were therefore faced with deteriorating buildings and having to travel further as schools were rationalised. By contrast, the costs of social security escalated in many countries, from around 8 per cent of gross domestic product (GDP) in 1979 to 13 per cent of GDP in 1996. The higher costs of social security tended to crowd out other areas of social spending such as health and education as governments sought to bring public expenditure under control.

The paradox seems to be that while there has been a sharp decline in employment, expenditure on manufactured goods has remained constant. This suggests that the decline in employment cannot be attributed to a shift in expenditure towards the service sector. Rather, there have been major productivity gains in manufacturing which can be attributed to the utilisation of new technology. According to the IMF, the decline in manufacturing employment needs to be explained in relation to major productivity gains in manufacturing rather than a decline in the manufacturing sector.

> An important implication of this discussion is that deindustrialisation is not necessarily a symptom of the failure of a country's manufacturing sector, or for that matter, of the economy as a whole. On the contrary, deindustrialisation is simply the natural outcome of the process of successful economic development, and is in general associated with rising living standards.[12]

From the perspective of the IMF, the loss of jobs in manufacturing does not represent failure, but is the natural outcome of development, of history, the utilisation of technology and progress. What is happening to manufacturing is what happened to agriculture a hundred years ago. Technology increases output and productivity, which requires fewer employees. Manufacturing output has not declined but the growth in manufacturing is no longer associated with growth in employment. Economic change does create winners and losers, with those in employment gaining from the new prosperity and the unemployed experiencing declining incomes. However, rather than governments seeking to protect employment in manufacturing through subsidies, tariffs or protectionism, the IMF argues that governments have no alternative but to live with the new realities of the market which, in turn, implies deregulation, reducing the costs of social protection and creating a more flexible labour market.

The IMF described the prospects for the world economy in 1997 as 'propitious', with inflation being subdued, a policy framework committed to price stability and fiscal imbalances being reduced with increasing determination. The IMF argument in brief is that growth prospects in the 1990s can be attributed to the commitment within nation-states to construct policies of price stability, reducing public sector deficits, which in turn are resulting in lower interest rates and higher investment.

On Europe the IMF points out that

> unemployment has risen further to new post-war peaks, and neither prospective growth nor the progress made with labour market reforms gives reason to expect any significant decline in joblessness in the near future. High unemployment and weak growth could make it difficult for EU members to meet the fiscal deficit targets associated with the plan for monetary union.[13]

The IMF argues that Europe can address the problem of unemployment by removing labour market regulations, which are a cost on employment, and making a commitment to a policy that reduces the costs of social security benefits.

> Mounting evidence that labour market regulations and high benefit levels are major contributing factors to high and persistent unemployment, excessive tax burden, chronic fiscal imbalances, and mediocre growth is too often ignored. It is therefore essential to strengthen the public's understanding of

the economic forces that are at work. At the same time, there is a continued need to persevere with comprehensive reforms to reduce the overly generous levels of unemployment compensation, tighten eligibility criteria, reduce taxes on employment.[14]

The IMF recommendations put the emphasis on the market and how to create flexibility within European labour markets so that the unemployed can be made more employable. The IMF answer is that Europe must reduce its labour costs by deregulating the labour market, removing regulations which make businesses less competitive and reducing social protection costs including unemployment benefits, pensions, health and education costs. By curbing these areas of expenditure, governments will reduce their deficits, reduce interest rates and reduce the costs to business.

Since the mid-1980s most European countries have sought to reform their welfare states. The attempts at retrenchment and containment of public expenditure have tended to have common elements. The major area to be targeted has been the social security budget with governments seeking to reform their pension costs or to restrict eligibility to unemployment benefits.

Wages and inequality

The globalised economy has also been associated with increased wage inequality between highly skilled workers and those with low skills in the advanced industrial economies. According to this thesis, the increase in trade between the developed and the developing economies has been concentrated in areas of production which require low skills. Because economies in the advanced economies cannot compete in terms of wages, jobs are being lost, or workers are being asked to accept wage reductions to remain competitive. Furthermore, because of increased competition and a squeeze on profits, companies in the advanced economies are switching away from production in areas of low skills to areas which require high skills, which provided higher rates of added value. This, it is argued, is depressing the wages of workers in low-skilled employment. In areas where the demand for high skills is on the increase, workers are receiving high rates of wages, which in turn are resulting in wage inequalities between skilled and non-skilled workers.

In contrast to the theory, much of the evidence would suggest that trade is the major explanatory variable. Trade between developed and developing economies only amounts to around 3 per cent of GDP, and trade has not been concentrated in areas of low-cost products.[15]

> Low-wage imports are simply not that important for most advanced economies, either in terms of quantity or their impact on domestic prices. Increased trade with developing countries therefore most likely accounts for only a small part of the increase in wage dispersion and the shift in demand towards high skilled workers.[16]

Another argument needs to be studied more carefully: that the expansion of trade has forced companies in the advanced economies to utilise technologies to replace low-skilled workers and therefore remain competitive. If a higher rate of technology replacement leads to lower costs in sectors where workers have low skills, there should also be an incentive to employ high-skilled workers with technology in order to reduce costs. The increase in wage dispersion in the 1980s and 1990s can be attributed to the utilisation of technology within the high-skilled sectors, which in turn have resulted in higher wage incentives as firms have sought to recruit key workers.

Implications for welfare

The implications for welfare systems are not immediately clear. Globalisation implies a reduction in the role of the nation-state, and the nation-state has been the foundation of much of what has happened in the development of welfare in the twentieth century. Deutsch sees the world system as a non-welfare state, and reviews the prospects for an international system.[17] But there are those who think that the trend to globalisation is fundamentally opposed to the welfare state: de Swaan has argued that the welfare state is at root a national phenomenon, and that it cannot be extended beyond national boundaries.[18] Jessop, in a striking phrase, refers to the 'hollowing out' of the state: although states have retained the appearance of sovereignty, in reality they have lost power both to sub-national regions and to international organisations.[19] There is increasing reliance on non-state organisations for the provision of welfare.

At the same time, the development of welfare systems at the level of the European Union is indicative of the potential for development of welfare on a much broader basis.[20] The problem which the Union has had has been to organise a strategy around the welfare systems of fifteen member states, each with established welfare systems and a range of priorities. This has been done in a number of ways. Much of the emphasis has fallen on 'harmonisation'. Slot identifies eight different patterns, including:

- the definition of law and policy at Community level;
- total harmonisation, in which rules are established from which no derogation is allowed;
- partial harmonisation, in which the only changes in rules concern people involved in cross-border movements;
- minimum harmonisation, in which minimal rules are outlined for implementation in different ways; the Commission refers to agreement on minimum standards as 'convergence';
- alternative harmonisation, in which different approaches and methods are described, and those who implement them are able to choose between them;
- mutual recognition of national rules; and
- mutual recognition of national control, so that each member state avoids making decisions in areas where another member state has authority.[21]

Although the European Union does not have the powers to develop a welfare state, it does have a social policy. Initially, the role of social policy was designed as an adjunct to economic policy, and was primarily concerned with the social consequences of moving to a single European market – promoting the movement of workers and capital, protecting the position of migrant workers, and offering funding to protect regions and industries in a state of transition. The Union has become, over time, progressively more interested in social policy in a wider sense: the Green and White Papers on Social Policy are concerned not so much with a set of policies as with a possible agenda for future action.[22] Much of the development of policy has focused on attempts to expand competence and the field of legitimate action.[23] In the case of poverty – which nominally falls outside the role of the Union – the Commission has attempted to develop a role in relation to intervention through the poverty programmes (in theory, a series of research programmes); through attempts to promote 'convergence' and the acceptance of minimum standards; and through the establishment of a role in relation to 'cohesion' and 'exclusion' as ways of justifying anti-poverty policy.[24]

The process of integration goes beyond harmonisation; there is an attempt to 'concert' policies across the member states, to bring them within a common framework. The strategy of the European Commission depends on the incremental development of the scope and coverage of systems of social protection.[25] Networks of social protection are progressively being extended, implying increasing interdependence and connectivity between people in different circumstances. As time goes on, networks of this kind – including pension provision and health insurance – can be expected to extend beyond and across national boundaries.

The European experience of integration is conscious and deliberate. Although there are other common markets – notably NAFTA – it is possible to see Europe as a special case. This means that the effects of globalisation are liable to be unstructured, and with the diminution in importance of national states it may happen that no one exercises any control. This is not a new scenario in social policy, because the indifference or impotence of national governments in the past has often led to similarly unstructured development. Those who are able to protect themselves – generally, those involved in stable economic processes – do so by gaining individualised rights; others are left out. The fragmented systems of Southern Europe are an example; there is strong protection for the privileged and well established (such as civil servants), and intermittent provision or exclusion for others.[26] The central problem for social policy, then, is the problem of exclusion.

Chapter 10

A new kind of society

Postmodernity

The idea of postmodernity depends on the idea that something which might be called 'modernity' came before it. The 'modern' period is generally understood as the period after the Industrial Revolution, though some people associate it particularly with the era of mass production, or 'Fordism'. The modern period is seen as a period of universal values and uniformity. Modernity gave ascendance to a view of progress and civilisation being founded in science and individual self-interest. According to McIntyre and Toulmin, modernity took a wrong turning by narrowing human potential to instrumental reason and the calculative individual, thus denying human creativity, romanticism and the aesthetic.[1] The world of the Enlightenment is portrayed as cold and individualised, where people take responsibility for their lives as individuals through hard work, thrift and self-help. The view that human progress was possible through knowledge and information has proved to be rather naive.

In the postmodern period, by comparison, society has become more fragmented, more diverse, more full of differences. This new context has been variously described as being 'postmodern' or 'post-traditional'. Postmodernity can be described as the process which seeks to replace the values of homogeneity and universalism with those of institutionalised pluralism, variety and ambivalence. Postmodernity is an attempt to deconstruct the role of language and discourse which in themselves create relationships of power. Within this context, White argues, there is a responsibility to disclose these relationships and so to reveal the nature of knowledge regimes.[2]

Postmodernity is based in a new 'consumer capitalism', which replaces the processes of productive capitalism. Lifetime jobs in consumer society are replaced by jobs which are based on knowledge, which force organisations to become less hierarchial. Individuals in a postmodern society now live in a world of knowledge and information which allows human beings to make choices about the life they would like to have. The pursuit of happiness becomes one of personal choice where happiness is no longer solely dependent on the material securities of housing, health and employment but also on issues related to quality of life.

At the same time, postmodernity reflects the break with the standardization of full employment and full-time work. Keynesian conventional wisdom pointed out that fiscal policy would generate employment through increases in demand and consumption. The break with Keynesianism has meant that the world of work is now less standardised; work is pluralised with the expansion of part-time working, contract work, flexible jobs and career breaks. Economic growth is not likely to achieve full employment; productivity in the service and manufacturing sectors is being achieved through the use of technology rather than expansion in the labour force. Consumer capitalism creates occupations which are part time, low paid and at the margin. The 1990s has been the age of wage reductions and of people working longer hours, despite high levels of unemployment. In Europe at present there are 18 million people out of work, yet those in work are working longer and for less pay. Unemployment continues to act as a threat to those in work who, despite reductions in living standards, have not shown any major resistance in the workplace.

This critique has to be understood at two levels: first, as a description of a 'socio-cultural form', a new kind of society and culture, and second, as a mood. Postmodernity as socio-cultural form refers to the structures and institutions which shape present-day society. One of the key concepts has been Foucault's understanding of history in terms of 'genealogy':

> a form of history which can account for the constitution of knowledges, discourses, domains of objects etc. without having to make reference to a subject which . . . runs in its empty sameness throughout the course of history.[3]

Postmodernity rejects the concept of the 'meta-narrative' – the attempt to explain everything.

Postmodernity as mood seeks to capture a climate of thinking that confirms a scepticism with science, with experts and knowledge systems. Postmodernity poses both opportunities for development and tensions. Some of the commentators involved outline implications for social policy, the politics of choice and policy making. These approaches are the subject of this chapter.

Post-traditional society

According to Giddens we now live in a post-traditional and post-scarcity society.[4] It is a society which is post-traditional in the sense that we live in a social condition which is not anchored in tradition, authority and institutions. Even if it is not a society which has completely broken anchor – it is at a minimum a society which has dragged anchor. A post-traditional society is therefore a society which is seeking to come to terms with uncertainty. Post traditional society is a society characterised by individualism but not the individualism as outlined in classical liberalism. The individualism of post-traditional society is associated with life styles and life politics. Individualism is now concerned with life projects, an emphasis on choice and autonomy which make life projects possible.

The concept of post-traditional society outlined by Giddens is one in which individuals are seeking autonomy.[5] While there is still a role for welfare, in the context of post-traditional society it has to be a form of welfare state which enables personal autonomy and choice. In seeking that personal autonomy, the individual becomes a citizen rather than a client of the welfare state.

The post-traditional society is also a 'post-scarcity' society, in the sense that in most developed countries, mass poverty is no longer an issue, and there are consumer goods available for the majority of the people in society. The pursuit of life projects in post-scarcity society involves the pursuit of happiness which cannot be counted in terms of the amount of taxes we are willing to pay and the collective goods we can consume. We have to calculate, for each decision we make about preferences, the utility derived from personal consumption and the income foregone to finance public goods. The happiness of post-scarcity society is achieved through inner dialogue, where the role of the state is to enable and empower individuals to gain that inner feeling of happiness. In this context the role of the welfare state should be directed to self-actualisation for each person. This is what Giddens calls a 'generative' welfare state, one which promotes the self-determination of individuals rather than focusing on the basic conditions of scarcity. The generative welfare state therefore is a welfare state that sees people as citizens or individuals who are unique and with their own life projects.

The supposedly 'new' social movements of post-scarcity society are described as being 'post-materialist'. Their primary concerns are not mainly with issues of redistribution of material resources but of uncovering forms of oppression, including patriarchy, institutional racism and the problems of a growth-orientated economy. New social movements associated with women's issues, problems of ecology and racial oppression are concerned with issues of space, of seeking to break with assumptions of homogeneity where inclusion has often implied hidden forms of oppression.

Tradition provided a moral and emotional binding of values that helped to create and reproduce community based on collective memory, history, culture and identity. By contrast, postmodernity points to a society that has broken with tradition and with those stories and narratives. Post-traditional society therefore is about the here and now: moral and emotional commitments are personal rather than collective; community is not assumed to exist but has to be constructed around redefined values. The present generation is increasingly removed from that collective memory and therefore their commitment to the welfare state is different from that of the generation which directly experienced the last war. There is now less of a feeling of a shared communal experience. Ideas on markets, individual self-interest and self-advancement are presented as new challenges and opportunities. By contrast, the generation which experienced the welfare state in the immediate aftermath of the war also knew what it was like to live with the market and the absence of welfare. The welfare state had an immediate impact on their quality of life. The present generation betrays the welfare state because it has never experienced life without the welfare state.

A third qualitative change in post-traditional society relates to the issue of trust. In traditional society, individuals trusted the guardians of tradition. These guardians included the church, philanthropic employers and professionals, including doctors and teachers. In post-traditional society the trust in these guardians is broken. The individual is now faced with competing expert advice.

There is no longer one message emerging from the guardians of knowledge and information. Instead information proliferates; it is also often conflictual and incompatible. The context is therefore one of increased uncertainty and increased feelings of individualisation, of having to choose between competing expert systems. For example, women who have reached the menopause can choose conflicting strategies like hormone replacement therapy (HRT) treatment or organic care; but HRT is associated with problems of blood clotting and organic treatment is still in its infancy.

Trust is no longer vested in guardians but in individuals. We now live in a world of 'as if' scenarios where each scenario is viable and plausible and where each community has its own interpretation of history. Although it is true to point out that human life has always been characterised by uncertainty, the new uncertainty of post-traditional society is founded on the growth of human knowledge. Rather than human knowledge leading to progress, as was argued by Enlightenment thinkers, the present levels of knowledge are creating new uncertainties. Rather than emancipation being dependent on history revealing itself through knowledge, emancipation in the context of postmodernity seems to depend on the ability of living with chaos.

The concept of post-traditional society creates a number of political and social challenges to the welfare state. There is the need to develop active trust – which means the opening up of the policy process to participation, increased transparency and accountability, thus making politics again a space of trust between experts and lay persons. This means removing those barriers which distort communication and creating openness and access to the policy process:

> In larger organizational contexts, active trust depends upon a more institutional 'opening out'. The 'autonomy' involved here can be understood in terms of responsibility and bottom-up decision making . . . Today, in many situations we have no choice but to make choices, filtering these through the active reception of shifting forms of expert knowledge; in such circumstances new forms of organizational solidarity tend to replace the old.[6]

The post-war consensus was founded on an exclusive agreement between those directly involved in production, which in turn denied citizenship to those individuals who were not directly part of that settlement. The settlement was relevant if you were a worker and less relevant if you became unemployed. Old age and sickness also contributed to exclusion. According to Giddens:

> The welfare state cannot survive in its existing form . . . the current problems of the welfare state should not be seen as a fiscal crisis but one of the management of risk . . . Such systems would have to escape from reliance on 'precautionary aftercare' as the main means of coping with risks; be integrated with a wider set of life concerns than those of productivism; develop a politics of second chances . . . and focus on what I have called a generative conception of equality.[7]

From the perspective of people involved in social policy, much of this reads oddly. Social policy is a practical subject, and the people with whom its practice is most concerned are not usually to be found grappling with the problems of a world in which scarcity has been forgotten. Giddens writes as if poverty no longer existed, we were faced with a new, almost unrelated set of problems, and we have moved to a concern with social relationships, like the problems of race and gender, because other problems have ceased to be important. This is a view taken by a number of right-wing critics on poverty, who hold that because the material problems of poverty have diminished, a concept based on inequality has been used to replace it.[8] Those of us who spend time in the study of poverty or who work with poor people see the world a little differently. Poor people are engaged in a constant struggle with scarcity. Their choices, their options, their life projects are circumscribed by their poverty. There is a 'web of deprivation', where people who pull themselves free from one strand can still be trapped by another.[9] None of this undermines the importance of the social relationships that Giddens is discussing, but it does raise important questions about the scope and validity of the analysis.

Postmodern ethics

According to Bauman:

> Postmodernity can be described as modernity emancipated from false consciousness, the post modern condition associated with institutionalised pluralism, variety, ambivalence,

contingency replaces the values of homogeneity and universalism. In contrast, post modernity can be perceived to be a new condition which represents the features which modernity sought to conceal; it unearths the hypocrisy of modernity – the false consensus – it seeks to deconstruct the language of power and reveal power.[10]

Ethics can be defined as a code of behaviour which is universal and which is applicable at all times. Ethics is about how human beings ought to treat each other at all times and, when something is wrong, it should be seen as being wrong at all times. The holocaust was wrong and it will always be wrong. By contrast, human beings produce behaviour which is often volatile and erratic and require rules which therefore have to have stronger foundations. These foundations have to be at a distance from day to day experiences.

Democracy reflects that erratic and volatile behaviour. Electoral politics can have dramatic effects on people's life chances. Electoral majorities provide political parties with political mandates that can change the status of citizenship and the right of residence for those who overnight find themselves defined as strangers and aliens. Arendt recognised the dangers of democracy and argued in favour of separating the social from the political. By including the social question of the welfare state into politics, Arendt argued that this would corrupt the political process.

Debating the future of the welfare state seems to be confined to arguments between a liberal and a communitarian view of the individual, issues of responsibility, rights and social justice. The concept of self according to a liberal view is the 'unencumbered self': the self who carries no baggage from the past, has no sense of responsibility to history but seeks to cut loose from communal roots and loyalties. The unencumbered individual lives within the universe of human rights, demanding the right to be treated as similar to other individuals and is perceived to be able to lift her or himself to a higher plane, detached, able to be critical and to move from the particular to the universal.

The communitarian view contrasts the concept of the unencumbered self to that of the situated self, that is, the self situated in the community where meaning and identity become possible only in the context of belonging, of solidarity and of responsibility to others. It is the sense of belonging that creates a sense of responsibility to others and to individual rights, and creates a context which makes justice possible. Welfare provision confirms the commitment to community because, through taxes, community and a sense of belonging is confirmed. It is the community that makes the individual possible. The individual has to be contextualised in history rather than being created as ahistorical, atomistic and unencumbered.

The postmodern ethic breaks with the liberal communitarian perspectives by suggesting that morality cannot be imposed. The argument that 'I am my brother's keeper' does not mean that 'my brother is my keeper', which is a basic premise of communitarianism. The morality I want to live by is not necessarily how the other interprets that morality. My view of justice is therefore personal to me, which means that I have to live with what is my yardstick as to what constitutes justice but also to acknowledge that others have a different view of justice. I might want to pay more taxes because I believe that it is likely to create a more equal and just society; the other might want to use charities as a means of focusing help on those in poverty. Postmodernity suggests that we cannot live with the morality as imposed by others or as others define morality. We cannot argue that our sense of morality lives at a higher plan to that of others, because we all have our sense of what is moral and what is just. We are each separate and unique; we are individuals, separated from others, yet we are at our best when we are with each other, rubbing shoulders but still remote, recognising the gaps but building bridges.

The morality of postmodernity is therefore the recognition of the bridges that individuals build to make the journey of life more enriching and worthwhile. The journey of life is an individual experience: we are born alone and we shall go to the grave alone. In between there is the journey of life, a journey that we share with others, but a journey in which we do not lose our sense that we are here primarily on our own. We are part of a community, but are also distant. We have our personal attributes or talents which we need to explore as we go through this journey – the framework that we create of institutions is one that makes the personal journey possible.

The welfare state seems to free us from that responsibility to others. The limit of that responsibility is defined by the taxes we pay. Taxation defines our responsibility to others; for example, we are encouraged to leave the caring of the elderly to the state and the professionals. My responsibility to my neighbour is defined by the state; my responsibility becomes my duty to pay taxes and this fills the void left by the lack of caring relationships. The welfare state therefore encourages separateness. Feminism, in seeking to secure the rights of women, is also implicitly saying that women should not take responsibility for their mothers or their fathers. Such a responsibility would stop them exploring their potential as unique individuals. Feminism indirectly points to relationships becoming contractual between men and women, women and their children, women and their parents. Women are involved in unpaid social reproduction, doing a job which is not their responsibility. In this sense therefore, feminism is truly postmodern.

The politics of the risk society

The concept of the 'risk society' points out that life experiences are to be explained in terms of risk. The risk society is atomised: it is individuals who take the risks. Individuals accept the risk of smoking since they know that smoking is a hazard to their health. Health professionals, having provided the information, argue that they should withdraw treatment from the individual who chooses to continue to smoke. The individual accepts the risk of smoking and therefore also accepts the responsibility for her or his own health. In a risk society, the state ceases to moralise about alcohol consumption. This applies equally to making provision for pensions, health care, sickness or education. In a risk society, individuals make choices based on information. The individual in a risk society does not need protecting by the state.

The risk society is, however, also about the disavowal of responsibility by government and business. Deregulated labour markets provide contexts where part-time workers have no access to sickness pay or rights to compensation against dismissal. In a deregulated labour market, the individual accepts the risks of living with competition. The employer has no responsibility to the employee outside the contract of employment. The risk society is unevenly experienced. The part-time workers, the manual workers and the sub-employed workers experience lower rates of pay than the full-time employees with high skills; they have fewer rights, and they are not unionised.

Disavowal of responsibility means that responsibility for the environment is left to the market. The market regulates the behaviour of potential polluters through tax penalties. The production of dangerous emissions becomes a risk for the individual who has to go through the courts to prove negligence. Ulrich Beck outlines a process of 'reflexive modernisation'.[11] He suggests that modernisation brings about dissolution of industrial society, because society takes a path which threatens its well-being. By contrast, reflexive modernisation is optimistic, because it argues for more experts, more knowledge, more public spaces and more dialogue. These create reflexivity and the potential of bringing about change, rather than a feeling of resignation and powerlessness.

The examples of economic growth and ecology illustrate the problems of reflexivity and powerlessness. The debate reaches an impasse because society is asked to make impossible choices between human progress and caring for the environment. Human progress is associated with growth, employment and economic prosperity. Those who argue a reduction in unemployment, less income inequality and more social justice are faced with the dilemma of favouring growth policies to deal with the problem of unemployment, in contradiction to a policy which seeks to protect the environment. The care of the environment is associated with taxation, the regulation of business and the inability of a country to compete in global markets. The risk society is therefore asked to make choices; people are presented with the costs and benefits and they vote for the political party that seeks to reduce the costs of the risk.

Both Beck and Giddens argue that the response to a risk society is to construct a climate of open government, served by expert advice, creating more trust and accountability in public institutions. Both are arguing within a framework of communicative rationality, as developed by Habermas; they believe that what is needed is improved dialogue and the creation of public spaces, which eliminates distorted communication.

The concept of a risk society confirms the shift from classical productive capitalism, which was founded on large-scale manufacturing, towards a consumer capitalism. The capitalism of the consumer society provides two faces. On the one hand there is the political economic sphere that provides for political legitimacy, providing spaces for participation and democratic accountability. On the other hand there is the techno-economic sphere that points to issues of the global economy and competitiveness. This consumer society points to the break with conventional politics and the decline of national politics in the context of the global economy. Ecological politics is not confined to national boundaries, since winds and weather which carry pollution do not know boundaries. Pollution produced in England kills forests in Sweden; fish farming creates imbalances on the sea bed. Cutting down forests alters the weather and creates problems of flooding. The politicians can no longer provide answers because the answers they seek are limited to national boundaries and the influence of national pressure groups. Beck argues for a new sub-politics, for the need to provide a regulatory framework which controls industry involved in risk, for a culture of self-criticism by professionals that ensures independence and separate advice, and for checks and balances through independent institutions with independent finance.

Living with the market creates a number of inconsistencies. The market is treated like an event which is beyond the control of the individual – the market cannot be bucked yet, at the same time, we live in an age when we want to be treated as unique individuals. The market by contrast creates feelings of isolation, individualisation and standardisation. Life events are considered to be personal failures. The negotiated family is made possible because both husband and wife are now in employment, which increasingly makes relationships voluntary and contractual. Couples stay together as long as they think the relationship is working, and both would be willing to move out of the relationship. Relationships are now more serial and individuals now accept that in a lifetime they are likely to be involved in more than one relationship. The welfare state also contributes to the negotiated family in that there are now a number of social policies which make it possible to leave relationships and set up independent households. The paradox is that in choosing such a strategy women are also becoming vulnerable to experiencing family poverty. The tendency is therefore towards differentiation of life styles. Although the existence of class cannot be denied, the attempt is to emphasise difference however marginal that difference. Clothing, the type of car, patterns of consumption make difference possible. Consumer society gives identity in terms of consumer goods.

The social meaning of inequality therefore also changes. The concept of the labour market reinforces the perspective that the experience of employment and unemployment becomes an issue for the individual. The individual is separated from others sharing the experience of unemployment. The loss of employment is not connected with macro-economic events but with the failures of the individual, the individual who fails to invest adequately in her or his education and training, the individual who prices her or himself out of the labour market because of high wages. Unemployment compensation is also based on individualised biographies. The unemployed are unemployed because of their own fault, and the solutions are sought in the individual characteristics of the unemployed people. The emphasis on the labour market ignores the possibility that when an industry shuts, creating large-scale unemployment in coal, steel or textile communities, the regeneration of new jobs within that community might take a generation. Instead, the market attributes the problems to the inadequacies of the people who are unemployed.

The idea of the risk society points to three aspects of individualisation. First there is the dimension of 'liberation' that points to the potential of individual emancipation, and civil rights. It points to the break with the politics of class and stratification and argues in favour of issues of plurality and difference, the independence of women and the emergence of the negotiated family. The second dimension relates to reintegration, when risk means living in the context of the labour market – flexible working where the individual experiences life as a personal biography. Reintegration in this sense takes place in the context of the individual in relation to a remote state where intermediate institutions, including trades unions, local governments and interest groups, are no longer avenues for collectivist action and reintegration into the state takes place in the context of individualisation. The third dimension of individualisation relates to the issue of political stability. The risk society points to the problems of living with class but also living in a world of consumer society where individuals emphasise difference through life styles.

The idea of the 'risk society' has appealed strongly to sociological thinkers who have been trying to update the Marxist paradigm. The language in which it is expressed – references to 'capitalism', 'immiseration' through risk, the dominance of the market, and the impotence of politics – reflects traditional Marxist perceptions. The spectre of terrors like pollution and food poisoning, the condemnation of capitalism for failing to offer material security and the emphasis on social atomization, blend middle-class anxieties with some of the traditional themes of the Socialist Workers'

Party, and the combination has about as much validity as its component parts. It should be obvious that most people's lives are not getting progressively worse, that society is not and never has been individualised, and that the market is not the only major social force at work. Perhaps less obviously, the Green buttons which are being pushed – about food safety, or the role of the market as a pollutant – also misrepresent what has been happening; food adulteration and public health are substantially less of a problem than they were in the nineteenth century, when the unregulated market truly dominated society.[12] Traditional Marxism ignored or belittled the importance of the interventionist welfare state; these analyses equally seem to be based on the idea that modern politics never really happened. The importance of the concept lies less in the situation it describes than in its understanding of what people may believe to be true. That is important in sociology because what people believe affects their behaviour, whether or not it is true. A society which is driven by concerns about road building, an obsession with *haute couture* and angst about biodegradable washing powder is not going to focus on the same kinds of issue which have engaged social policy in the past.

Postmodernity and the individual

The representation of individualism in postmodern society is ambivalent. On one hand, postmodernity can be seen as an atomised society, in which the bonds which hold people together are dissolving. This is the view of Ulrich Beck, who sees the process as a reflection of postmodern capitalism. Beck's thesis of individualisation relates specifically to a changing economic context – that is, from classical forms of capitalist production to a capitalism which is more directed at consumer society. Classical capitalism was accompanied by identities around industrial communities including steel, coal or textiles, and a welfare state directed at identifiable households. The capitalism of the globalised economy creates a society of individualised biographies of individual risks rather than collective biographies and histories.

> 'Individualisation' means, first, the disembedding of industrial-society ways of life and, secondly, the reembedding of new ones, in which the individuals must produce, stage and cobble together their biographies themselves . . . Both disembedding

and reembedding do not occur by chance, nor individually, nor voluntarily, nor through diverse types of historical conditions, but rather all at once and under the general conditions of the welfare state in advanced industrial society.[13]

This form of individualisation is not based on free choice, but people are condemned to individualisation – the project of individualisation is therefore based on compulsion.

At the same time, postmodernity has the potential to be liberating. The dissolution of traditional bonds represents an opportunity as well as a challenge. The attempt by men and women to construct personal biographies and individual histories means that, in future, relationships will no longer be held together by status-based marriage rules about duties of men as breadwinners and of women and motherhood. Women in the 1990s need to think about education and personal careers if they want to live independent lives.

> These models do not weld people together but break apart the togetherness and multiply the questions. Thus they force every man and women, both inside and outside marriage, to operate and persist as individual agent and designer of his or her own biography.[14]

Bauman has argued that the most important discovery of post-modernity has been the issue of freedom – freedom in the sense that we have come to increasingly accept, that there is no one right answer but that there are different interpretations of the same text. This means that we are increasingly forced to negotiate, to compromise and therefore to recognise the other. Quoting from Odo Marquard, Bauman points to the implications of breaking with the concept of one truth:

> If – regarding a holy text – two interpreters, contradicting each other, assert I am right, my understanding of the text is the truth, and a truth imperative for salvation, it may come to a fight. But if they agree instead that the text can be understood in a different way, and if, this is not enough . . . they may start to negotiate – and who negotiates does not kill.[15]

Within the context of the new freedom therefore the process is to make explicit and transparent the nature of consensus. Bauman argues that what keeps us alive is the right to disagree and to dissent and it is that living with dissent and with uncertainty which creates the major challenge.

> Consensus and unanimity augur the tranquillity of the grave-yard (Habermas's perfect communication: which measures its own perfection by consensus and the exclusion of dissent, is another dream of death which radically cures the ills of freedom's life) it is in the graveyard of universal consensus that responsibility and freedom and the individual exhale their last sigh.[16]

In postmodern society, life politics replaces the emancipatory politics of modernity. The emancipatory politics of modernity gave prominence to emancipation from traditional struggles against exploitation and to demands for more social equality. Life politics by contrast is more related to individual life projects, demands for self-actualization and personal identity.

> The capability of adopting freely chosen lifestyles, a fundamental benefit generated by a post traditional order, stands in tension not only with barriers to emancipation but with a variety of moral dilemmas.[17]

Demands for gay rights, equal opportunity policies, policy commitments on harassment – all pose major challenges to welfare institutions both in relation to the treatment of clients but also in relation to employment, selection and training. Recent specific examples include challenges to racism and sexual harassment within the police force.

The welfare state has seen a move to individualism in both senses. On the one hand, welfare systems have increasingly come to depend on individualised circumstances. The particular rights which are established in most of continental Europe depend on the work record and earned rights of each person; for others, the welfare state has become increasingly means-tested and focused on those in need. On the other, welfare policies have increasingly been concerned with pluralities. In the context of an individualism which is founded on personal autonomy, self-actualised lives and on individuals striving to make sense of their biographies and personal life styles, the twin issues of difference and equality become central.

The claim that we are different, unique individuals with our own personal life projects gives primacy to the commitment of the right to be different.

Difference and equality

The welfare states of the post-war period sought to promote homogeneity and assumed that the communities which were served were also homogeneous. Welfare and citizenship were defined in the context of homogeneity. Provision was based on a specific view of life styles. Men went to work whilst women stayed at home and looked after children. The insecurity of unemployment affected men and it was therefore men who had to be adequately insured against the risks of unemployment, ill health, injury and cycles of interruptions from work. Insurance for men was based on the assumption that men would claim the relevant benefits on behalf of their family. This was based on a further implicit assumption that families were stable and durable and, furthermore, that family breakdown was a problem for a small minority. Families, it was assumed, would stay together, children would be cared for within the context of the family and the family would provide support for older members. These assumptions were not sustained purely because of ideological reasons since these views also carried practical advantage for government. Reliance on the family contributed to the control of public expenditure. If women could be provided for within the context of the family, the benefit received by men could be seen as providing for all dependents.

However, as Connolly has pointed out, the language of homogeneity is a strategy for containment. It continuously needs to point to the outsider, to be ghettoised and used on occasions as the 'other'.[18] This 'other', which includes the migrant, the unemployed youth and the single mother, resists assimilation into the discourse of homeogeneity, because assimilation often means the need to reject the past – to surrender identity and biography and become part of community. Community is constructed. It is based on a series of myths and beliefs on collective memories and histories which then become the boundaries of the 'imagined community'. The 'other' is indispensable to the imagined community because these groups provide the discourse of contrasts. The identity of the 'in group' is sustained through the devaluation of the other. Neighbourhoods are no longer places of stability but of continuous influx of new faces. The neighbourhood has the potential of defining who are the insiders and the outsiders, establishing stereotypes of the neighbourhood and the strangers. Strategies can seek to include or exclude – the first assimilates whilst the second merges all strangers as aliens, as outsiders. Policy practitioners involved in dispensing public provision at a local level respond to strangers by confirming separateness. At local government level, politicians and administrators come under pressure to sustain separateness. There are frequent accusations that local authorities have developed ghettos for people in ethnic minorities. In the age of strangers, the strangers are defined and constructed by the welfare state.

To illustrate the tensions between equality and difference Hannah Arendt utilised the twin concepts of the Parvenu and the Pariah.[19] The parvenu seeks to be accepted by the homogeneous community and accepts the policy of assimilation and seeks to be assimilated within the framework of the imagined community. The continuous attempt to please, the denial of oppression and discrimination result in the denial of self, of personal dignity, culture and history because the aim is to live within the history of the neighbourhood. The parvenu seeks to become part of the neighbourhood, preferably to vanish and melt rather than continuing to stand out as the stranger. The aim of the parvenu is to make a success of her or his personal biography, to succeed according to the criteria set by the neighbourhood. The migrant has to be sure that the decision to leave has had a positive result. By contrast, the pariah (in Arendt's sense of the word) gives priority to the right to be different, to be accepted as being different, and therefore to be accepted as the other. The pariah questions the strategy of assimilation because assimilation denies self. Furthermore, the pariah asks whether the community is real or imagined and whether the values which underpin that community are shared. To the pariah, all individuals are pariahs, seeking to establish their uniqueness and difference. But the stranger is asked to be assimilated because of being the stranger. The pariah draws strength from being separate – neither denying nor apologising for being different, but insisting on the uniqueness of individuals as a universal phenomenon.

Postmodernity, by contrast with the homogeneous approach of the welfare state, seeks to give primacy to difference and pluralism. The assumptions of homogeneity and the attempt to create agreements have often resulted in producing false consensus, which has often implicitly generated forms of hidden oppression and intolerance. The right to be different is therefore assumed to be a form of celebration since it breaks with homogeneity and creates opportunities and chances for the human being to be treated as a unique individual with individual life projects. This idea of the individual with rights to individual life projects means that individuals need to be defined as different and unique and to deal with issues of hidden hypocrisy not previously questioned. The world is made more transparent and forms of suppression are made explicit. However painful, child abuse, violence against women in the home and racial and sexual harassment need to be recognised as existing rather than denied and hidden.

Within postmodern theory, the right to be different is combined with a specific approach to equality. Equality and difference are combined to suggest that laws, rules and procedures are needed to provide a framework for equality. This framework also allows individuals to confirm difference. Women can choose to live separately and to live alone with their children, to seek a new relationship with a man or another woman, to embark on employment, professional careers and studying – projects which have always been available to men. In the context of family breakdown, of women electing to leave relationships rather than to stay and of relationships becoming increasingly serial with children being brought up outside their original family, the system of income support has to change to reflect societal change. To make these life projects possible, women therefore demand support from the welfare state. For women to work there has to be a system of childcare which is available at low cost and which is flexible to the working hours of women. Women need to be given the opportunity to work more flexible hours, the opportunity to break through the glass ceiling in career opportunities and to have access to finance to enable them to return to study.

Recent debates in Europe and the USA on the condition of single parents and policy commitments on 'Welfare to Work' confirm conflicts and confusion of policy making. Policy makers are at one level seeking to moralise about the family and single mothers whilst at the same time seeking to confirm their commitment to the individual. The language that is emerging seeks to connect the costs to the taxpayers and provision of benefits for single mothers. It is a language which provides politicians with a moralising crusade on the family and about single mothers. Remoralising the family is used as a strategy to make benefits for single parents increasingly dependent on means-testing whilst at the same time reducing the amount of benefit being paid. In Connolly's terms, single mothers are used as the other, to be contrasted and devalued in the context of the imagined community.

There are major problems for welfare states when the attempt to respond to the difficult problems of treating people equally but differently. The commitment to difference, plurality and diversity points to procedural justice, of written constitutional rules that commit public institutions to transparency and accountability. Individuals who experience institutional racism and other forms of oppression which create social disadvantage, exclusion and marginalisation need avenues and pathways which ensure the rule of law.

This represents an important challenge for communitarians. Differences need to be celebrated, but the celebration of difference itself creates new problems. As the imagined community seeks to celebrate its collective history, that celebration often means the oppression of the other. A clear example has been Northern Ireland. When the Protestant community celebrates its tradition, and marches through Catholic areas to confirm its historical rights, the Catholic community in turn feels oppressed. The 'other' may seek in response to join diasporas, where the individualised experience of being an exile is dissolved into a shared and collective experience. The new diasporas have been built around labour, culture, disability, even the status of victim. Their growth shows increasing resistance to homogeneity. However, these forms of resistance are often perceived as undermining and threatening community. The question is how and who is defining the imagined community that results in the exclusion of the other.

Postmodernity and politics

Christopher Norris has argued that the concept of postmodernity and its central claim that there is no such thing as truth has created a political vacuum which encourages a feeling that anything goes, that all is relative and that we live in a plurality of scenarios. There is no single text to understand and interpret, but a number of texts which are being interpreted in different ways; social policy reflects that plurality of viewpoints. Within this plurality, debates on issues of poverty and social justice are given equal status to issues of self-interest, markets and fashion. Postmodernity celebrates that we live in the world of signs and simulation. It confirms a climate where there is no longer any difference between myth and reality. It is a world which comes to favour conservative politics, a politics of pragmatism and the end of ideology. Typical examples have been the criticisms levelled at Lyotard and Foucault and their non-committal approach to politics and the possibility of emancipation and social justice. Both authors have argued in favour of keeping their academic writings separate from their political practice. Whilst Foucault has been criticised that his writings encourage a disillusionment with politics, biographers of Foucault have pointed to his involvement with radical social movements.

> I think I have in fact been situated in most squares on the political checkerboard, one after another and sometimes simultaneously: as anarchist, leftist, ostentatious or disguised Marxist, nihilist, explicit or secret anti-Marxist, technocrat in the service of Gaullism, new liberal, etc . . . It's true that I prefer not to identify myself and that I'm amused by the diversity of the ways I've been judged and classified.[20]

The postmodernist approach to politics downgrades the importance of class and gives ascendance to the individual. Postmodernists are sometimes represented as radicals: the advocate of postmodernity seeks to deconstruct the language and discourse of the professionals and to disclose issues of power. The postmodernist questions the false consensus of homogeneity and points to the problems of exclusion. Conversely, postmodernity has been criticised, for example by Peter Taylor Gooby, for its tendency to undermine the radical analysis of society.[21] If there are no class relationships, if the role of ideologies is undermined, and if there is no politics, there may be no scope for social policy.

Chapter 11

Explaining social divisions

Social divisions

There can be a considerable social distance between people in the same society – for example, between people in upper and lower castes, between different linguistic or religious groups, or between people of different races. In the nineteenth century, Disraeli wrote famously of Britain as having two nations, the rich and the poor.[1] This was giving much more than the view that rich and poor people were in different positions; it was saying that rich and poor people had such an economic and social distance from each other that they lived their lives separately, had no direct social contact, and had virtually different cultures. In extreme cases, the divisions in a society can be so strong that the society itself falls apart – the position, for example, in the former Yugoslavia, where religious and ethnic differences were expressed in civil war and partition. In most circumstances, however, we tend to talk about social divisions in a much more restrained way. Typical examples are the divisions of class, gender, race, poverty and age. These are, properly speaking, aspects of inequality rather than examples of division in themselves; they do not preclude social contact between the groups. However, there are circumstances in which people in these segments of society can be taken to inhabit different spheres – that is, different aspects of social life are reserved for some people rather than others. So, although women are not kept separate from men, there is still a remarkable degree of segregation in occupational activity: there are jobs for men, and jobs for women, and the jobs for women tend to pay less.

The examination of social division is central to critical social policy, which refers to the structure of inequality as both a major set of issues in its own right and as a central mode of explanation for the development of social policy and the social services. Although much of this analysis has been shaped in Marxist terms, much has not, and in recent years there has been a progressive extension of critical analysis to consider different intellectual sources, and different forms of structural explanation.

Critical theory

The most appropriate starting point for understanding critical social policy is probably 'critical theory'. This is not a very clear term; there is no canon or critical theorists' manifesto to which one can comfortably refer and, although the term obviously refers to a set of related approaches, there are striking differences in the work of writers who might be referred to as critical theorists. The term originated in the work of the Frankfurt School, who fused Marxism and insights from philosophy and psychology. The Frankfurt School is now sadly neglected, though some of the ideas they put forward are still fascinating and, even when they are flawed, are provocative and unsettling. Adorno suggested that racism finds root in a particular psychological type which divides up the world into structures of authority.[2] Erich Fromm argued that the hierarchical structure of some societies related not simply to social forces but to the psychological urges to dominance and subservience.[3]

Although the writers of the Frankfurt School saw their work as an alternative to Marxism, it was still strongly influenced by Marx. The main elements which distinguished their arguments were, first, a critical (or disapproving) view of the social structure, based in normative judgments about that society. Although critical theorists, and notably Habermas, have emphasised issues of personal autonomy, it would be as true to say that the criticisms of society have centred on issues of inequality, power and oppression. Second, critical theory applies universal values, taking a view from outside the society; there is a presumption of equality, because arguments are taken to apply consistently to everyone.[4] Third, critical theory depends on a moral commitment to the use of knowledge about society in order to bring about social change. It stands, on this basis, in contrast to the positivist social science which was fashionable in the middle of the twentieth century (though not, one should note, to much of what has been done in social science since).

The theorist who is most worthy of note in this is Jürgen Habermas. His writing is sometimes difficult, but he is engaged in a difficult enterprise: the construction of a rationalist theory which can be used for a normative examination of society. Habermas writes with a thoughtfulness and rigour which put some of the other writers considered in this chapter to shame. Although Habermas writes from a standpoint broadly sympathetic to Marxism, and uses much of the Marxist terminology, he has distanced himself from many of the specific conclusions of Marxism. Habermas expresses reservations about, amongst other things, the assumption of a materialist base in society, the dominance of economic considerations and productive relations, the determinism of historical materialism, and the role of the state. There are reservations to make about the arguments which Habermas tries to put in the place of Marxism – the idea of the 'legitimation crisis', discussed in Chapter 3 – but in many ways the present chapter is based in the kind of critical enterprise which Habermas has put on the agenda.

Power and social control

The emphasis on power is one of the defining features of radical thought in the analysis of society and social policy. 'Social control' is used to point to ways in which power is exercised over people. This is a slippery idea, which is used at different times to refer both to the operation of social norms – rules which govern, for example, restraints on violence or child abuse – as well as mechanisms through which state action favours a dominant class.[5] From a Marxist perspective, it is clearly the second category which is important and distinctive about capitalism, though Marxists have been happy to draw on examples from social norms when it is convenient to do so. Examples include, for example, the sanctions put on people who fail to maintain themselves and their families, the suspension of rights to benefit for failing to work, or the harassment of social security claimants by the authorities. New technologies have resulted in surveillance, self-regulation and self-policing. Closed-circuit television on the high streets, grilles separating civil servants from social security claimants, payment through banks and the use of computers in dealing with clients of the welfare state have all contributed to extreme feelings of individualisation in relation to the powers of the state.

There are instances which can be given of the direct use of control but those which are available are ambiguous, because often the wider public accepts the legitimacy of the position. Criticising people who are out of work may seem to be peculiarly in the interests of employers, but in any society there is an expectation that people will contribute to society, and in Soviet Russia 'parasites, tramps and beggars' were subject to public sanctions.[6]

The maintenance, or 'reproduction', of the social system is determined through hegemony.[7] Hegemony is a process through which social perceptions and values are shaped, influenced and ultimately determined in favour of the dominant class. Bourdieu suggests a number of ways in which the education system preserves hegemony and reproduces the social system.[8] It maintains it by educating and training the labour force. It reinforces the class structure by stressing the division of labour and continuity of occupations between generations. It socialises people into the dominant culture and the virtues of the political order. Feminists have added another important point: that it educates people into sexual divisions.[9]

Since the demise of intellectual Marxism, analyses of social policy which are concerned with the uses of power are frequently referred to Foucault. Foucault has interpreted a series of issues, including the control of mental illness and the uses of punishment, as an expression of the exercise of power. He sees power as 'a multiplicity of relationships of force which are inherent in the domain in which they are exercised, and which make up their organisation'.[10] Power is the dominant force in society: 'power is everywhere, not because it embraces everything, but because it comes from everywhere'.[11] Foucault makes a series of propositions about power:

- power is not a simple relationship, but is so complex and manifold that it cannot be avoided;
- power relationships are inherent in other types of social relationship;
- power comes from below as much as from above: it is socially constructed;
- power relationships are not subjective; and
- power implies resistance.[12]

In some parts of Foucault's work, power appears to be essentially disciplinary in its nature, achieving outcomes through the control of deviant behaviour; at the same time, his emphasis in his writing on sexuality falls on social control through more subtle means – the establishment of a dominant culture and ways of behaving in a society. He refers to this combination of dominant norms and physical control as 'bio-power', a term which has appealed to a range of writers, including feminists. Bio-power controls the smallest aspects of social behaviour by constructing views and codes of conduct which affect how people understand and use their bodies.

The core of the analysis, and the terms in which a Foucauldian analysis of power tends to be referred to, depend on the analysis of power in terms of discourse. Foucault's contribution has been to point to the potential power that is embedded in language and policy statements, a form of power that hides and denies oppression, discrimination and exclusion. The analysis of language confirmed the changing nature of suppression and surveillance.

> In every society the production of discourse is at once controlled, selected, organised and redistributed by a certain number of procedures whose role is to ward off the powers and dangers, to gain mastery over the chance events, to evade its ponderous, formidable materiality.[13]

The deconstruction of language points to an attempt to understand the dynamics of power and domination as constructed through language – the analysis of the language of policy documents and policy statements seeks to make explicit assumptions which are often implicit. Deconstruction is therefore essential in analysing assumptions that policy makers have about the family, the unemployed, people in poverty and groups of young people who are increasingly seen as being alienated from the dominant discourse.

> These reevaluations draw attention to (among other things) problems associated with the growth of the welfare activities of the modern state. They recognise that, however benevolent these activities may be in intention, the discourses and institutions that emerge with them often promote a deep and progressive disempowerment of their clients.[14]

Foucault's approach to the policy process is that individuals become involved in local struggles, local not in the sense of geography but in relation to a specific discourse, against specific forms of oppression and the abuse of power. Examples of such local struggle include movements for the rights of prisoners, the civil rights of workers to join trades unions, the demand of patients for greater transparency of the medical profession and the rights of single mothers against surveillance. Within a Foucauldian framework groups involved in highlighting civil rights, the abuse of power by the state and public sector institutions represent the attempt to create an alternative discourse to that which is presented as universal and natural.

Foucault identifies different kinds of social control – the adoption of dominant norms, the imposition of sanctions and the control of deviance – as reflections of similar social phenomena. This is a tenable position, even if it sits oddly with the emphasis elsewhere in his writing on the diversity and lack of structure evident in social processes. The main weakness in the argument lies in the view that power is everywhere, which is either false or vacuous. If power is taken to mean that social conditioning underlies everything we do, it is virtually empty – true, but not very informative. If power is taken to mean the exercise of control in the context of a structured social relationship, and Foucault's proposition is that every kind of social relationship reflects this kind of power, it is false – an absurd reduction of the field of human experience, whether it is going to a party, walking on a beach, playing cards or listening to music, to a single kind of influence. If the statement is moderated and confined to the analysis of power itself it is more useful, but it is still not exactly the sharpest of tools. It does not distinguish between the operation of social norms and the situations in which one group in society might act to exert power over another. On the same basis, it also fails morally to distinguish between legitimate and illegitimate forms of social control. Preventing the sexual exploitation of children and incarcerating women who demonstrate for equality are not equivalent, and it is not necessarily helpful to argue that they are.

It is difficult to refrain in a section discussing Foucault from reflecting on his extraordinary contemporary influence: a series of books have now been published which explicitly outline the analysis of social policy in Foucauldian terms. Foucault's many enthusiastic fans think that he is independently minded, unprecedentedly insightful and original. Others find him woolly and slapdash. Part of the difference is explained by the uneven quality of his writing: *La volonté de savoir*, which is the first volume of the *History of Sexuality*, is much better written than *Surveiller et punir*, and much clearer about his intellectual approach and concepts. Foucault is never fully explicit, however, about his intellectual framework. He is woefully ignorant of the insights and arguments of anthropology or the sociology of deviance on the subjects he writes about, which means he never tests his ideas against contradictory views and observations. He keys into Marxist terminology, but makes no attempt to use the terminology – or any other kind of language – rigorously. Despite his emphasis on the importance of history and genealogy, his attempts to present history are often overtly schematic. His historical research combines sweeping generalisations and a disregard for contradictory evidence with very questionable interpretations of the events he selects. For example, Foucault's dependence on the idea that transformations of behaviour marked the change to bourgeois society is difficult to sustain. The assertions that punishment gave way to technological surveillance during the nineteenth century,[15] or that madness was tolerated in preindustrial society[16] – observations are central to his analysis of these subjects – are just not true. Little of what he writes about mental illness stands up to serious examination if you happen to know anything about the treatment of mental illness (and Kathleen Jones, who knows rather a lot about it, has written a devastating critique[17]). Given the deficiencies, the weight given to Foucault in sociological study is difficult to understand.

Oppression and empowerment

Thompson defines oppression as 'inhuman and degrading treatment of individuals or groups; hardship and injustice brought about by the dominance of one group over another; the negative and demeaning exercise of power.'[18] This identifies two essential features of the concept of oppression; first, that it is something done by oppressors to people who are oppressed; and second, that it relates to the use of power. It is debatable whether either of these is enough in themselves to constitute oppression: bullying in a school playground, for example, is negative and demeaning, and causes great suffering and distress, but it is not normally thought of as a form of oppression. Equally, treatment can be oppressive even though it falls short of being inhuman or degrading; an example is the exploitation of illegal workers. What is missing is the sense that oppression takes place within a structured relationship of power – which is why employment is oppressive in circumstances where bullying is not.

The idea of 'oppression' owes much to Marxist analysis; it was one of the key terms used by Marx himself, referring to relationships in which people exercised power over others and were able to exploit them. Freire's work on community education in developing countries gave the term a new vigour as a means of referring to people who were downtrodden and disadvantaged. Freire referred directly to the Frankfurt School (particularly to Fromm); he saw oppression as the antithesis of 'humanization', characterised principally by freedom and autonomy. His particular contribution was not so much an analysis of society as the identification of a strategy for countering the imbalances of power found in the Third World through collective action.

> The starting point for organising the programme content of education or political action must be the present, existential, concrete situation, reflecting the aspirations of the people. Utilising certain basic contradictions, we must pose this existential, concrete, present situation to the people as a problem which challenges them and requires a response – not just at the intellectual level, but at the level of action.[19]

In recent years, the concept of oppression seems to be enjoying a renewed vogue, especially in the context of social work studies, where it has been taken to refer to the consequences of power without necessarily identifying any particular structure of power.

> British society is saturated in oppression . . . of black people by white people, working class people by middle class people, women by men, children and old people by 'adults', disabled people by able people, and gay people by 'straight' people.[20]

The idea of 'anti-oppressive practice' has been gaining ground in social work, and a number of texts refer to it.[21] Anti-oppressive practice, Dalrymple and Burke argue, 'is about minimizing the power differences in society'.[22] The methods they propose include collective work; setting achievable goals; using policy/legislation; being informed; strategic positioning (that is, placing oneself in order to have maximum effect for one's clients); and a strong and positive position in relation to adversity. This is pretty limp stuff: no one is going to argue that social workers should be ill-informed or should set unattainable goals. Strategic positioning and effective advocacy are part and parcel of mainstream social work. Only one of these methods – collective work – seems in any way distinctive, and that not by much. Anti-oppressive practice seems to have more to do with maintaining the correct political stance than with changing what social workers do.

There are two main problems with the idea of oppression. The first is that it is very, very wide; if middle-class people oppress working-class people, men oppress women, and adults oppress children and old people, then most of the population is oppressed. If oppression is a general experience, the concept does not do a great deal to separate the sheep from the goats. The second problem is that it is not very clear how the oppression is manifested. It is one thing to say that women, racial minorities or old people are disadvantaged, about which there is not much argument; it is another entirely to say that this is the result of oppression. Oppression implies that disadvantage is produced by a structured power relationship. That calls for an account of the structure of power, the process by which disadvantage is produced, and a description of how the power has been exercised to produce the disadvantage. This sort of account is hard to find. Many commentators tend to take evidence of social control or structured inequality as if they constituted evidence of the exercise of power, which they may not be. Social control is often evidence of social norms rather than power; the production of disadvantage is not proof of intention. Inequality can usually be explained without reference to power at all. People start out with differences in their endowments, possessions, social relationships, education and life chances; it would take an exercise of power to alter this so that people were not disadvantaged.

Patriarchy

Feminism has been represented as an 'ideology', but there is more than one kind of feminism. 'Liberal feminism' is basically liberalism as it applies to women, emphasising the principles of individualism and equality of respect; 'Marxist feminism' is largely based in the application of Marxism to the particular situation of women, though many Marxist feminists have recognised the deficiencies of traditional Marxism as an explanation of women's position. The most distinctive form of feminism, and one which does have a distinctive claim to be an ideology in its own right, is radical feminism.

Radical feminism operates a critical perspective in its combination of condemnation of the status quo – the disadvantage of women as a class – with a moral position: that women should be able to live and act autonomously.

Radical feminism begins from the premise that gender is fundamental to social relationships. The basic relationship is one of patriarchy: men oppress women. The term 'patriarchy' was popularised by Kate Millett:[23] Juliet Mitchell describes it as 'sexual politics whereby men establish their power and maintain control'.[24] The structure of power invests men with power which is reinforced through a system of social norms and explicit and implicit sanctions. Radical feminists have pointed, for example, to women being incarcerated or classified as mad because they did not submit to their husbands or did not wish to marry. Firestone argued that it was women's biology which made them vulnerable to domination in these terms; this view is not generally shared by other feminists, who are much more likely to see women as an oppressed group. Delphy refers to women as a 'class':

> the concept of class . . . puts social domination at the heart of the explanation of hierarchy . . . Class is a dichotomous concept and it has, because of this, its limitations; but on the other hand, we can see how well it applies to the exhaustive, hierarchical and precisely dichotomous classifications which are internal to a given society – like the classification into men or women.[25]

Radical feminists have argued that the hierarchical structure of power between men and women vitiates relationships between individual men and women; some have gone so far as to argue that the patriarchal nature of society makes equality impossible.

The concept of patriarchy has been criticised by Michèle Barrett, a Marxist feminist, on the ground that it is much too general.

> The resonance of this concept lies in its recognition of the transhistorical character of women's oppression, but in this very appeal to longevity it deprives us of an adequate grasp of historical change. How useful is it to collapse widow-burning in India with 'the coercion of privacy' in Western Europe, into a concept of such generality?[26]

Barrett tried initially to argue that the term should be reserved for societies in which older men dominated others, but subsequently accepted that patriarchy might be a useful shorthand for a general position. Her initial argument, though, is worth considering. The general view of patriarchy identifies all men as members of the oppressive class, and all women as oppressed; Barrett's proposal recognises at least that some men are relatively powerless.

The basic proposition that power in society tends to be held by men is not difficult to accept, but several problems remain. First, there is the general problem of trying to explain disadvantage in terms of oppression. The construction of society to the advantage of one group is not the same as the statement that such a group exercises power. The position is often unclear, because people who have power may find that other people change their behaviour to win their approval. Where norms are generally accepted, it is impossible to say with any confidence who is responsible for the oppression. Widow-burning and female circumcision are often carried out by women, not by men. Second, gender is not the only factor which governs the distribution of power in a society: other factors include race, class and status. Lesley Doyal comments that the 'white, western, middle-class domination of feminist theory and practice' has been breaking down in recent years, primarily as a result of the diverse contributions of women from different kinds of minority. The comforting view of women as a single class, unified by a common experience of oppression, is not tenable.[27] Third, if there is a problem in trying to represent 'women' as a whole class, there is equally a problem in trying to present 'men' in these terms. Delphy's assertion that the supremacy of men over women is 'exhaustive' should not be allowed to stand; it means, if taken literally, that no men are relatively powerless relative to any woman, which is nonsense. If women and men have varying degrees of power and influence, then the classes are not hierarchically ordered, but overlapping.

Feminist arguments have played a large part in the development of writing about social policy in the last fifteen years or so. Much of the analysis has focused on three areas: the role of women as carers, their dependent status in the family, and the impact of the division of labour in the household on women's resources and poverty. By contrast, work on health and education relating to social policy has been relatively limited, which is the result of academic demarcations rather than lack of interest. The study of health and education have been dominated by the sociology of gender, which tends to focus on social relationships and issues, rather than administrative processes and responses.

Writing on feminism tends to switch between individualistic and radical premises. Writing about the position of women in the family is highly individualistic; Payne writes about the 'poverty and deprivation women experience within affluent households'.[28] This treats women as if they were completely atomised, or divorced from any society, and played no part in the household. Their use of heating, food, furniture or household goods is treated as irrelevant. This is, no doubt, comforting to female academics who want to think of themselves as members of the ranks of the oppressed, but it lacks conviction. A stronger use of liberal arguments can be seen in criticism of the 'glass ceiling', which prevents women rising in organisations. The premises behind this are liberal – they depend on arguments for equal opportunities, not equality. This implies that people must have equal opportunities to be unequal, and that if women as a group do not have the same degree of inequality that men have it is evidence of disadvantage or discrimination. Liberal feminism is not enough, however, to account for these arguments; the basic interest in the position of women as a group depends on the kind of collective or class-based perspective which is exemplified by radical feminism.

At time the arguments lead in opposite directions. Pascall – recognising the ambivalence – criticises the welfare state both for its invasion and direction of the private sphere and for its failure to intervene, which leaves women dependent on men.[29] This reflects a tension which is typical of feminist writing: whether women are to act and be treated as autonomous individuals, or as members of a society. In practical terms, there are liable to be similar contradictions. Pascall criticises the assumption that women are primarily responsible for childcare[30] while emphasising the particular importance of child support for women, because 'their responsibility for children, for caring and maintaining, tends to continue, whether or not men provide'.[31] This reflects the problem of deciding whether policy and analysis should deal with the world as it is, when women are often dependent and disadvantaged, or as it should be, where women have a relative degree of independence and equal status.

Overview: a stand against injustice

There is much in these positions to agree with: society is riddled with injustice, and people are treated in degrading and demeaning ways. Unfortunately, people who take these positions rely on others agreeing with them, and they do not always take the trouble to say what they mean clearly, unambiguously and sensibly. There are lazy arguments, in which whatever happens is assumed somehow to have been the result of design or deliberate policy, without any mechanism being visible through which this might have been done. There is a tendency in some arguments to damn or dismiss any policy: anything beneficial is a subtle form of control, while anything negative is proof of malign intention. And there is often a besetting pressure to conformity in argument, in fear that contrary views will support the Enemy, which means that writers try not to be too rude about silly ideas if their authors have their hearts in the right place. Readers may perhaps have noticed that some of the comments in this chapter break that particular rule. People who are disadvantaged need advocates who are better than the advocates for other groups; good intentions are not sufficient reason for sloppy thinking.

Part 3

New challenges to social policy

Chapter 12

Society

The impact of a changing society

If society is changing, the relationship of people to the society they live in is also liable to change. This may seem obvious: people live and die, and their relationships are not fixed. At the same time, some of the theories that have been considered depend on the view that the structure of society remains the same, despite change. A river moves constantly, but it can move without changing its course very much. Marxism views certain elements in capitalism as fundamental, and argues that society is characterised by the same relationships as it was a hundred years ago. Individualists who are opposed to the very idea of society argue that what seem to be social movements are merely the results of interaction between individuals.

Against this one has to set a range of views: there have been unquestioned changes in the structure of family, community, the industrial process, economic alignments and so forth, which affect the rights and responsibilities which people have towards each other. The question as to whether these affect the basic structure of society is virtually impossible to resolve, but for our purposes it does not matter very much: whether or not things have changed fundamentally, what really matters is what is happening to the pattern of social relationships, and what this implies for policy.

Individuals in society

There is a popular myth of 'human nature': that people do not change. Even in radically different cultures – like Evans-Pritchard's study of the Nuer,[1] or Ladurie's stunning recreation of fourteenth-century France[2] – there are some recognisable patterns governing the relationships between people, families and communities. This consonance, though, is deceptive. In the first place, our own culture has many features derived from different influences: there are still identifiable elements of paganism, tribalism and feudalism, even if these elements are minor relative to others. Second, there is a tendency to understand or reinterpret historical situations in different cultures or societies in the terms of our own.

The perception which people have of human nature depends strongly on the society of which they are part. The Christian doctrine of 'original sin' was gradually supplanted by the Enlightenment view that we were a blank sheet to be written on, a *tabula rasa*. The view that some people are born inferior, a powerful element in many societies (including, in the twentieth century, the Nazi era) is in conflict with the liberal view that people are born equal and must be allowed the potential to develop. The Victorian concept of human nature, which is still important today, held that our nature, like that of the rest of the animals, was individualistic and competitive; against this, socialists and collectivists have argued that our nature is, in fact, collaborative. (The belief that nature consists of lots of animals going their own way is false, and there are very strong counter-examples – like the Portuguese Man of War, a 'colonial animal', which consists not of one animal but a multitude which behave as if they were a single entity. In the nineteenth century, Herbert Spencer argued that people in society were individuals who lived in a constant state of conflict with each other. It was Spencer who coined the phrase 'survival of the fittest', later used by Darwin to describe the mechanisms behind evolution. Peter Kropotkin, now generally remembered as an anarchist thinker, challenged Spencer's individualist assumptions, arguing that it was as false in biology as it was in society.[3] There is an interesting point here, apart from the question of what is natural and what is not: it is that the way we understand problems in science is often shaped by what is going on elsewhere in society, because it influences what people imagine and what they think possible.)

If personal identity is constructed in the light of social relationships, people change with a society. The social construction of the individual shapes the way we think, the way we express ourselves, even our physical reactions. In the Introduction, we discussed a highly socialised view of the nature of the person – in Wrong's view, an 'oversocialised' concept.[4] If people have to be understood in a social context, it is the social context, rather than the organism, which defines the person. The implications of this may seem extraordinary. One consequence is that it is possible to be a person without being human. In law, a company or corporation can also be a 'person'; companies can own and dispose of property, they can be insulted, and they can take action. The converse is that it may be possible to be human without being a person. Miller and Gwynne, in the context of a critical discussion of residential care, write about 'social death'.

> To lack any actual or potential role that confers a positive social status in the wider society is tantamount to being socially dead. To be admitted to one of these institutions is to enter a kind of limbo in which one has been written off as a member of society but is not yet physically dead. In these terms the task society assigns – behaviourally though never verbally – to these institutions is to cater for the socially dead during the interval between social death and physical death.[5]

The terms in which the idea is stated suggest that they are writing about social death as an analogy: lacking roles is 'tantamount' to death. From a sociological viewpoint, the argument can be put more strongly; people who are left without roles are not persons any more, which means that they are socially dead. (The converse may also be true; people who have died may continue to have a social presence, affecting the way that people after them behave.)

The most obvious practical applications of this approach lie principally in individual casework rather than in social policy in the broader sense. Although there is an approach to individuals which is based on their internal and private psychology, such psychodynamic approaches are questionable in approach and their efficacy: non-directive counselling has never been validated.[6] Compton and Galloway describe a process through which a picture of a person's social life, identity and relationships can be built up from people and situations around that person as a means of identifying possible routes for maintaining circumstances or fostering change.[7]

There is, though, a more general issue: that society does, in important ways, construct the nature of the individual. This is central to some of the arguments that were considered in Part 2, notably Foucault's arguments about the social construction of sexuality, and feminist arguments about the pervasiveness of gender. Both of these positions imply a moral consequence: that things do not have to be that way, and that what society has done can be undone. These arguments are radical, in the sense that they go to the root not just of social relationships but to what kind of being we are. By comparison, the arguments in social work which suggest that people's behaviour can be changed seem almost modest, but they are no less important. Society makes people, and it can make them different.

Families

Changes to the family are a key element in the concerns expressed by many critics about society. The current trend, widespread in Europe and America, is for families to be impermanent; a high proportion, though not a majority, are broken by divorce. Childbirth outside marriage is increasing, though much of this is accounted for by couples in relatively stable relationships who may become married at a later point. The growth of illegitimacy and the breakdown of marriages affect the upbringing of children and, consequently, the reproduction of society in the broad sense – the transmission of norms and values through the family as the primary unit of socialisation. Particular concern has been expressed that the trend to fatherless families disadvantages children[8] and exposes mothers to dependency.[9] Further, the corollary of families without fathers is that there will be fathers without families. The association of illegitimacy with crime, which has been the subject of several right-wing attacks on single parenthood, may seem far-fetched but it has its roots in the belief that families are a basic element in socialising, and a concern about what young men are doing when they are marginalised in the family and in society.[10]

There are two distinct trends to unpick here. The first is the impermanence of marriage as the basis for family life: the effects of cohabitation before marriage and divorce are indicative. This might well have effects on children's upbringing – Dennis and Erdos review the evidence[11] – but its influence is confounded by the second trend, which is a strong association of family instability with economic factors. There is a strong link between unemployment or economic vulnerability and the formation and duration of marriage. There are links between marital dissolution and unemployment, whether the unemployment precedes the marriage or happens during the marriage.[12] Cohabiting parents are likely to be on very low incomes, and cohabiting fathers are particularly likely to have been unemployed.[13] Research in France also shows an association between a marginal position in relation to the labour market (referred to in France as précarité, or sub-employment) and instability in marital relationships; at the same time, some criticism has been made of the indicators used to measure the effect.[14] In relation to responsibility for children, there is higher illegitimacy among people who are poorer, and a greater demand for residual childcare.[15] Murray has noted a correlation of .85 in the UK between the distribution of unemployment and the growth of illegitimacy.[16] (It seems important to note that this does not support Murray's contention that an increase in illegitimacy is 'the best predictor of an underclass in the making';[17] the association may indicate other things altogether.)

Rodman offers a plausible explanation of the connections. He argues that the economic circumstances of poor families shape their domestic organisation and, in particular, their gender roles.[18] The reaction of women is central to the analysis. economic marginality of poor men means that although they can at times fulfil conventional social roles, they cannot do so consistently. If men are to be 'breadwinners', they need to earn money; but a central characteristic of poor people is that their income is liable to interruption. This, Rodman believes, changes the position of men relative to women. The woman cannot rely on the man as a breadwinner in the long term. A man who is not earning becomes a drain on the family's resources; the woman has to be prepared to jettison him. However, even if there is an economic incentive to drop the man, there is still a social incentive to have a partner. Poor families, and poor women, share the aspirations and values of higher social classes. A common adaptation is to move through a sequence of partners – 'serial monogamy' rather than promiscuity – as the woman finds different men to act as partners and sources of support. This clearly does not square with dominant values, but it is identifiably an adaptation of such values. For the most part, Rodman argues, people in lower social classes share the norms and values dominant in the rest of society. Other things being equal then, they will act in much the same way as the rest of society. But other things are not equal. Rodman describes the process of adaptation as a 'value stretch', in which poor people do not actually reject dominant values but 'stretch' them to fit their situation.[19]

Rodman also extends the analysis of the effect of marginal employment on the family to consider relationships with children. Families have to be centred on mothers rather than on either fathers or on both parents jointly. At the same time, a common experience of the poor families he studied was that the interruption of income left them little able to support their children; this meant that farming children out to relatives and friends was fairly common, which also implies in turn the necessity to reduce the strength of the emotional ties between mothers and their children. (There are examples of this in Britain, but it is not so visible as to be a major factor in child-rearing. At the same time, it may reflect on some issues in relation to childcare for the poorest families.)

William Julius Wilson's work follows, apparently independently, a similar line of argument; he identifies a shortage of 'marriageable' or economically stable males, and comments that 'the increasing inability of many black men to support a family is the driving force behind the rise of female-headed families'. His main conclusion is that male joblessness has to come high on the policy agenda.[20] Jencks argues that there is no association between the rise in single parenthood and the size of the marriage market, as proposed by Wilson. The pool of marriageable males among African Americans has remained stable, but single parenthood has increased.[21] This shows that if there is an African American underclass in these terms it is not necessarily growing, but it does not show that the processes which are being described are not taking place. Jarrett, speaking to African American single parents, records similar attitudes which tend to confirm the general concern.

> 'Right today I'm right glad I did not marry him because he still ain't got no job.'
> 'If we get married and he's working, then he lose his job, I'm going to stand by him and everything. I don't want to marry nobody that don't have nothing going for themselves . . . I could do bad by myself.'
> 'I got to see a place where he's helping me. But if you don't help, I got no time.'[22]

This kind of adaptation to economic and social circumstances is described in the ethnographic research of Sullivan and Anderson,[23] both of whom are concerned with the consequences of an early initiation into sexual activity. The patterns of behaviour are adaptive because they reflect adaptation to circumstances. It might be argued that limited economic prospects are associated with an early end to education, because the returns from education are few; there may be an early push to independence because neither parents nor children have reason to prolong support.

This offers a model of considerable explanatory power. Illegitimacy and serial monogamy are often treated as 'immoral' behaviour, which means that circumstances associated with poverty are likely to attract moral condemnation. The reaction of other classes to this behaviour may then be to blame the poorest for their circumstances.

Communities

Changes in communities are harder to identify than changes in the family, because the very idea of a community depends on the establishment of some kind of relationship. The term 'community' is used to mean so many things that it is difficult to say whether it really means anything at all: a famous paper by Hillery identifies ninety-four different meanings, and the only thing they have in common is that they are all about people.[24] The literature on community is also often tinged with a degree of sentimentalism, and complaints about changes in the community sometimes seem to be part of nostalgia for a bygone age rather than a comment on any specific changes in society.

Community can refer to social networks, to people with common interests or culture, or to people in a particular geographical area. When people bemoan a 'loss of community', it usually means a breakdown of social networks within a geographical area – for example, because the population has changed, because families and young people move away, or because the area becomes impoverished through economic decline. These issues are most evident in poor areas (a term which some individualists have disputed, arguing – quite wrongly – that it must refer to a physical concentration of individual poor people).[25] A poor area is an area in which there is a constellation of social problems and deprivation; they have poor housing, a run-down environment, a lack of security and low status. Poor areas are formed through a process of residential segregation. Wilson argues that people with the capacity and resources to move to more desirable locations do so, leaving behind those with lower resources;[26] at the same time, there is a process of selection in the condition of newcomers, who (like those who have become homeless) may be unable to exercise choice in the market, or who may be unable to command sufficient resources to choose a more desirable area. Massey, Gross and Shibuya argue, by contrast to Wilson, that there is relatively little out-migration; what there is is high mobility among those who are poorest which, when combined with the restricted opportunities for relocation, tends to lead to movement towards greater segregation.[27]

There is nothing new about poor areas: the same kinds of problem were described by Charles Booth in his research in Victorian London (Booth called them 'poverty traps').[28] The issues which have emerged have been identified with certain related problems – in the USA, with the issues of race, in France with the creation of the suburbs, in the UK with the failure of certain public housing estates.[29] The root connection is the problem of poverty: that people with the least resources are those who are least able to choose, and the magic of the market brings them together in the places which are least to be chosen.

It is more difficult to decide whether social relationships within neighbourhoods can have some effect on individual behaviour, though the implication of the argument in the section above on individuals is that they must. Crane examines 'neighbourhood effects' on school drop-out rates and teenage pregnancies. He reviews several studies, controlling for family incomes, benefit receipt, religion, race, educational attainment and so forth, before presenting his own data; the effects of the neighbourhood seem to be large.[30]

The class structure

Changes in the economy have been discussed in an earlier chapter. In this section, it is important to note only that the workplace has important implications for social relationships; it is a major source of social identity and social contact. Workplaces have changed significantly with the movement from manufacturing to service industries and the growth of clerical work; some writers see the growth of teleworking, which moves work from a dedicated workplace into the home, and flexible hours, as having considerable potential for social change. The implications of such changes remain speculative. The most obvious development in recent years is not so much the change in the workplace itself as the absence of work for a significant proportion of the population.

The idea of the 'underclass' is associated by some commentators on the left with some of the anti-welfare literature from the USA.[31] A common line of attack has been that the category is meaningless:

> 'Underclass' is a destructive and misleading label that lumps together different people who have different problems . . . the latest of a series of popular labels . . . that focuses on individual characteristics and thereby stigmatises the poor for their poverty.[32]

Gans, similarly, argues that

> the term has taken on so many connotations of undeservingness and blameworthiness that it has become hopelessly polluted in meaning, ideological overtone and implications, and should be dropped.[33]

But the abuse of a concept, and its association with politics we disapprove of, is not a very good reason for supposing that it has no value. If the same criteria were applied generally in social science, there is hardly a concept that would be left standing.

The idea of the underclass was intended to point our attention to an area which was all too frequently left out of conventional class analysis; the term was first used on the left, not on the right.[34] Many of the people with whom social policy is concerned are not working class in the traditional sense; in relation to the most commonly used classifications they are not really in any class at all. Discussion of the underclass provided a means of conceptualising the position of many people with which social policy analysts have centrally been concerned.

The problem with this kind of approach has been the way that it has been abused by right-wing critics prepared to condemn the poor for their poverty. The kind of attack which was commonplace in the 1960s has resurfaced in full flow.[35] Auletta associates the underclass with 'violence, arson, hostility and welfare dependency', and Murray with 'drugs, crime, illegitimacy, homelessness, drop-out from the job market, drop-out from school and casual violence'.[36] In the UK, the *Sunday Times* has flogged the issue remorselessly:

> The underclass . . . is a type of poverty: it covers those who no longer share the norms and aspirations of the rest of society, who have never known the traditional two-parent family, who have left the official labour force for good, who are prone to abuse drugs and alcohol at the earliest opportunity, who do poorly at school and who are quick to resort to disorderly behaviour and crime.[37]

The element of moral judgment has tainted the debate, and it makes it difficult to discuss the issue without being vulnerable to the accusation of blaming the victims. But the problem is not, as Matza pointed out, the terminology which is used: it is that people in the lowest strata of society are generally stigmatised, and any term which is used – the 'abyss', the 'submerged tenth', the 'hard to reach' and so forth – becomes over time a term of abuse.[38] There is nothing in the term underclass which is inherently insulting, and it is usefully descriptive: it refers to a group of people at the bottom of the class structure. The central problem is not what they are called; it is that they are at the bottom.

A 'class' of people is defined, sociologically, as a group identified by virtue of their economic position in society. The underclass is composed of people whose economic position is not simply poor, but effectively excluded from the mainstream of economic production.[39] The underclass are a class, in the formal sense, because exclusion defines a set of economic and social relationships. A Marxist class analysis defines people's class in terms of their relationship to the means of production; there must then be some distinction between the proletariat and those who have no direct relationship to the industrial system. A Weberian approach would reinforce this distinction, though it might also suggest a number of underclasses rather than one homogenous group. The Registrar-general's classification of occupations starts from the significant premise that status groups are primarily defined in terms of occupational categories, and it follows that those with no occupational category are likely to fall below the levels occupied by those who have. The underclass is a socio-economic grouping which falls beneath the criteria by which other socio-economic groups are classified.

Bulmer has argued that we need, as a counterbalance to individualistic theories, 'a structural theory of the underclass which locates the phenomenon in its social context'.[40] The central argument for viewing the underclass in structural terms is that people in it have a distinct economic and social position. The term does not describe a single, cohesive group; most analyses of poverty emphasise the diversity of problems which people experience. There is no reason to suppose a common culture, shared values or any form of class consciousness, and Wilson stresses the importance of social isolation (or atomisation) as opposed to a 'subculture'. What poor people share in common is a social and economic position – that they are relatively powerless, of low status and socially rejected. Rodger is not convinced that this is enough to constitute a class in the formal sense, but he does refer to 'a substructural space in society for the unemployed which marginalises them'.[41]

The experience of people in the underclass is not uniform, and it is possible to distinguish at least two main economic categories – which might, in Weberian terms, be taken to represent two different classes, though the dividing lines are not clear. One group contains those who are genuinely excluded from the labour market altogether, and so are financially dependent. This group includes pensioners, and many disabled people. Those who are dependent and outside the labour market are not only economically marginal: they are in breach of social norms by virtue of their lack of contribution to society.[42] The simplest explanation for their lack of status is the failure to reciprocate, though there are other sources of prejudice and rejection.

The second group consists of people who are not simply excluded, but who have a marginal position in relation to the labour market. These include single parents, some disabled people, and many people with low employment status or skills, any of whom may find themselves employed only casually, intermittently or for limited periods of time. The experience of 'sub-employment', referred to in the discussion of the changing economy, is one which produces a distinctive economic position:[43] people are marginally and intermittently employed, and economically precarious. This is also the sense in which Morris and Irwin have taken the concept of the underclass,[44] identifying a distinct set of patterns of marginal employment.

There is a case to say that the underclass consists not of people who are poor, but of those who are most vulnerable to poverty through the process of exclusion. People in the underclass are likely to have to depend on benefits at some point. However, many of those who depend on benefits do so only for short periods – there are transitions through unemployment, serious illness or single parenthood – and it seems inappropriate to identify the underclass too closely with a dependent population. There is the potential for people who are marginalised to contribute, though when they do contribute it is often by work with low status and rewards. It is possible to view this group either as being hier- archically in a slightly preferable position to those who do not work at all, or alternatively in a distinctive social position.

People who fall within an underclass differ from others because their economic position is different. Their earning power, even when work is available, is limited, and their resources are irregular and insecure. Benefits which are tied to the labour market – like national insurance, which relies on an unbroken contribution record, or benefits for people on low incomes – often disadvantage the claimant whose employment status is marginal. Benefits which presume a stable set of circumstances – like benefits for single parents, or pensioners – are claimed if, like the cases of pensioners or people with dependent children, the circumstances can be taken to be stable. But they may not be claimed if, as in cases of single parenthood, of benefits tied to accommodation or of recurrent sick- ness or unemployment, the situation is not stable.

If, besides, the kind of analysis which identifies sub-employment and economic marginality is correct, then people in the underclass are specially vulnerable to this kind of instability – which implies, in turn, that they will be particularly vulnerable to policies which assume that they will live in one place, have one form of employ- ment, have one partner and have clear continued responsibility for dependents. It seems likely that the degree of transience is produced by the very shortage of resources which leads to support being required. This is particularly important for policies for benefits, where it is difficult to respond to changes in conditions as they happen – which is the central assumption behind a number of benefits, including benefits for unemployment, benefits for single parents, and means-tested benefits.

The dependency culture

The idea that the welfare state has fostered a 'dependency culture' has resurfaced in recent years. This is a revival of a very old criticism of social welfare, not a new one. Benjamin Franklin wrote of the situation in England in 1766 that:

there is no country in the world in which the poor are more idle, dissolute, drunken, and insolent. The day you passed that Act [the Poor Law], you took away from before their eyes the greatest of all inducements to industry, frugality, and sobriety, by giving them a dependence on somewhat else than a careful accumulation during youth and health, for support in age and sickness.[45]

Herbert Spencer was making the same case a century later. Economic evidence about the Poor Law is equivocal, but it seems fairly clear that when work was available, people became employed and avoided the Poor Law, and that when work was not available, they did not. This is a hoary old myth, which blames the poor for their poverty.

The idea can be separated into two parts. The first is the argument that the provision of welfare acts to undermine the incentives and willingness to work of people who are poor. Charles Murray's analysis of the underclass offers a clear example. He argues that the different patterns of behaviour among the underclass are primarily explicable in terms of rational economic choices. Much of the critical literature on his work[46] has concentrated on the accuracy of the observed material, but what is most striking about Murray's case is not the misuse of material but how little he relies on such evidence at all. He uses the example of a fictional couple, Harold and Phyllis to explain why a family which is on benefit might become locked into dependency on welfare benefits. Murray begins with three premises:

1 People respond to incentives and disincentives. Sticks and carrots work.
2 People are not inherently hard-working or moral. In the absence of countervailing influences, people will avoid work and be amoral.
3 People must be held responsible for their actions.[47]

Harold and Phyllis behave according to supposedly rational rules of human conduct, not as others have behaved in similar circumstances. The conclusion that welfare fosters dependency, though Murray tries to emphasise the sophistication of his analysis, follows from these premises quite straightforwardly: if people are paid for doing nothing, they will choose to do nothing, and they must expect to be blamed when they make that choice.

The premises are questionable at best. The proposition that people respond to incentives and disincentives is true by definition; if people do not respond to a measure, then it does not have an incentive or disincentive effect. If, however, the purpose is to argue that people are motivated in fact by financial sticks and carrots, and solely motivated by such means, the proposition is much more debatable. In the first place, people's responses to financial impetuses vary; the generalisation is usually justified at the aggregate level in economics because differences cancel each other out. The idea that people respond to incentives directly is plainly wrong; the concept of 'inelasticity' indicates that even if responses are proportionate to incentives, it may take a very considerable spur to alter choices and preferences. Second, the assumption is that other things are equal. There are costs and benefits to be weighed, and the economic costs of being poor, unemployed or a single parent are considerable. Third, financial motivations are only one kind; people have other motives for their actions, including moral, social and psychological factors. Eithne McLaughlin's work on the motivation of unemployed people shows that it is not true that people will only work if they have an increase in income; that the source of income matters as well as its amount; and that women's behaviour in any case reflects a different pattern of constraints, requiring choices not between work and leisure, but between paid and unpaid work.[48]

The argument would be on stronger ground if it were presented, not as a general proposition about individual behaviour, but as an economic proposition concerned with aggregate behaviour. The main economic issue is that, as incentives change so the behaviour of some people changes, which leads to a trend in a particular direction. That is the basis for all economic arguments about incentives to work. Murray relies in addition on the proposition that there is a set of incentives which apply peculiarly and uniquely to people dependent on benefits. This is at least defensible; the 'poverty trap' is an illustration. What is not clear is whether the financial arrangements actually do have very much incentive or disincentive effect. The evidence which exists on incentives to work is equivocal.[49] Some individual effects have been demonstrated, most markedly on women whose partners are not working.[50] However, the structure of incentives depends as much on the structure of the labour market as on the benefits system, and aggregate figures do not show any association between benefits and participation in the labour market. Because unemployment is primarily related to economic activity rather than social security benefits, there is no relationship apparent between the relative generosity of benefit systems and the levels of unemployment prevailing over time.

Murray's second premise is bizarre. It is probably not true that people are 'inherently' hard-working or moral, but then we have already argued that people are not inherently anything. If this is intended as a general statement about the way people are, it is plainly wrong – most people do work for a substantial period of their lives. As for the statement that 'in the absence of countervailing influences, people will avoid work and be amoral', it is directly contradictory to the first premise – which must mean that people will work and be moral if there are incentives to do so. Since work generally yields some marginal economic benefit, and moral conduct is conceived within a set of reciprocal social networks,[51] there are such incentives, and it would require countervailing influences to stop them working. The idea that people will not work if they are paid benefits has to be wrong, because most people of working age do work even though they might be paid benefits instead. The problem is that Murray has treated benefits as the only incentive people have to determine an outcome; for the argument to apply, people would have to be paid for doing nothing and also face the situation where there is no economic or social benefit to be gained by working and no sanction for not working. This could be true where the work is for wages which are as low as benefit rates, and benefits are withdrawn at a rate of at least 100 per cent against marginal earnings; it could only be true for the poorest sector of the population. Hence the concern that poor people are particularly vulnerable to the 'disincentive' effects of benefits. But the force of the second statement seems, then, to amount to little more than the force of the first.

This is evidently not Murray's intention. The second premise reads more on the face of it as an assertion about original sin than it does about economic incentives. This element is strongly linked with the third premise – that people should be condemned with bell, book and candle for succumbing to the siren temptation of a life of ease on Aid to Families with Dependent Children. It is not really necessary to make any judgment about this, because it serves no obvious purpose in the argument. If you believe that people's motivations are solely financial, then moral condemnation is not going to make any difference and, if you don't, then an extended analysis like Murray's argument on Harold and Phyllis, which completely ignores the moral and social dimensions, starts to look perverse.

The second proposition in the idea of the 'dependency culture' is that welfare has led people to be persistently poor, creating an underclass. This is the basis of the kind of condemnation reviewed in the previous section. The proposition is not supported by the available empirical evidence for a very simple reason: poverty does not last in the way that critics have supposed. Individual dependency is generally periodic,[52] the constitution of the dependent population below retirement age is not stable,[53] and the population of the underclass is constantly changing;[54] the apparent persistence of poverty does not describe continuing poverty among a constant group of people.

The decline of the moral order

Although the discussion of social order can quite legitimately be taken to refer to the mechanisms through which people engage in collective social action,[55] this is not what people are concerned about when they complain that the fabric of society is under threat. This expresses the general concern that social relations are deteriorating, that violence and antagonism are increasing, that society is threatened with disorder. The president of the National Association of Head Teachers writes that 'Society is fragmenting and teachers are struggling to fill the vacuum left by parents, the church and law and order.'[56] Gertrude Himmelfarb writes that 'the moral equilibrium seems to have been lost',[57] linking the problems to fatherless families, welfare dependency and crime. Some of the feverish representation of these issues in the media has been described as 'moral panic', but that does not mean it is not important. Moral panics are representations of people's moral perceptions, and they cannot be dismissed so lightly. It may not be true that there is a huge amount of satanic abuse of children, or attacks by dangerous dogs, but is it the quantity that matters? Any case gives reasonable cause for concern.

Like many other popular myths, the perception of moral decline is half true. If there were no truth in it, and no evidence could be called in its support, no one could ever take it seriously; conversely, if there were no reason to doubt it, no one would. The evidence which seems to suggest a deterioration of standards points to growing levels of divorce, increases in violent crime and sexual offences, problems of drugs and violence in schools, and the physical deterioration of the urban environment through graffiti, litter and vandalism. There has certainly been, in Britain and the USA, a rising trend in serious crime. The growth of economic problems reinforces the view that crime is rising, because crime and disorder seem to have some links with economic problems, though the relationship is not straightforward. Steven Box, reviewing evidence from Britain and the USA, finds a complex relationship between rising crime and economic recession. There is some support for the idea that unemployment and serious crimes (other than murder) are linked; much more clear is the link between crime and income inequality, which emerges from most studies in the field.[58] At the same time, crime cannot be understood solely in these terms – in Britain and the USA, reported crimes have increased substantially in the post-war period. Some of the factors which give the impression that crime is rising are, however, based on a limited view; some are pointing to particular problems of modern times; some are misconceptions.

The first point is that perceptions of crime are not necessarily proportionate to its prevalence. If people become less tolerant of a crime, they will report it more often – which means that an improving situation might produce a greater number of crimes. This is arguably what has happened in relation to rape. Crimes of property become more apparent when people have property to steal, and when householders are insured against theft (which requires them to report the crime). Domestic violence is, regrettably, still largely invisible.

Second, as society changes, so certain types of crime become more prevalent, while others are less prevalent. Crudely speaking, stealing cars is only possible where there are cars, offences with firearms are only possible where firearms are available, and drug abuse depends on the particular situation where certain drugs are both available and illegal. By contrast, highway robbery appears to be less common than it used to be (travellers are less likely to be isolated and vulnerable), bigamy now seems quaint rather than consummately evil, and rustling is difficult in the middle of New York or Paris.

Third, we are not necessarily comparing like with like. Many crimes are committed by young males in their teens, but the effect of prolonging education through the teens is that they are now found in school rather than at work. The problems of the urban environment have to be balanced against other developments – the growth in developed economies of the suburbs and the hinterland of cities, the use of high-density housing, and the growing problems of waste (although the problems of litter are pretty trivial when compared with the problems of disposing of night-soil from the rookeries of the nineteenth century).

Jock Young describes three main current approaches to the study of crime. 'Left idealism' argues that crime is pervasive, and generated by social inequalities. It emphasises the tendency for crime to be exaggerated, contrasting the stress put on the visible crimes of the poor rather than on the relatively concealed crimes of the rich. 'Administrative criminology' sees crime as opportunistic, and so as avoidable or preventable, rather than being rooted in deep-seated social concerns. 'Realism', on both the left and the right, emphasises the growing rates of crime; the right-wing attribute the problems to the moral breakdown of society, the left-wing to the injustices of an unequal society.[59]

It seems important to contrast the gloom and despondency of some 'realists' with other features in society – the growing material prosperity of developed countries, progressive improvements in health, or the extension of social protection. The perception that society is disintegrating is a myth, but it cannot be discounted on that basis. On the contrary, myths play an important part in politics; Sorel uses the idea of the myth to emphasise the importance of such perceptions in framing beliefs and forming policy.[60] If people believe something to be true, Thomas and Znaniecki famously argue, it is true in its consequences.[61]

Overview

Despite everything that has been written and said about the effect of a changing society, much of the material covered in this chapter is depressingly familiar. The supposed issues – such as moral decline, the threat to the family, the degeneration of the cities or the dependency culture – are all old ideas, which have been on the agenda of social policy for a couple of hundred years. The main positive developments relate, in strategies against exclusion, not to a new problem but to a new way of thinking about old problems. In some cases, notably in relation to the dependency culture and the negative arguments about the underclass, the arguments persist despite overwhelming evidence to the contrary, which indicates that they have more to do with ideological perceptions of the provision of welfare than they do with any serious analysis of society.

Chapter 13

The economy

Social policy and economic policy

Social policy has been to a large extent dominated by economic policy, because economic policy determines the amount that government is prepared to spend. In some places, notably the Federal Republic of Germany, this ordering has been done explicitly: the Müller–Amack report in the 1940s argued for the primacy of economic policy as a means of furthering social welfare. But the same calculations are made in other countries. In the UK, the reform of government in the 1970s made it possible to restrain public expenditure on welfare within strict budgetary limits established by the Treasury. Attempts to conform with the criteria for European Monetary Union have led to major constraints on welfare spending in France and Italy – or at least, attempts to do so.

The discourse which tends to be in the ascendant within finance ministries is that social policy has to be financed by the private sector economy. It is the economy for goods and services produced within the market which produces the real wealth and that therefore social policy is the attempt to redistribute that wealth once it has been created. This represents the primary concern of government as being to create an economic framework that ensures the creation of wealth before making decisions on social policy. Social policy represents consumption and that consumption cannot happen without production. Social policy also connects with economic context since social policy decisions inevitably represent expenditure which needs to be financed. The costing of social policy is therefore related to resourcing of different social programmes and priorities. Governments might make a number of policy statements on universal rights to health and education but such statements remain rhetorical until they are resourced and turned into policy realities through making decisions on expenditures, taxation and insurance costs.

It has been part of conventional wisdom to point out that economic prosperity has been the enabling factor in financing developments in social policy during the first two decades of the post-war era and, equally, that economic stagnation has explained social policy retrenchment in the 1980s and the 1990s. Periods of economic growth result in higher levels of employment and higher tax yields to government through tax on disposable income and consumer expenditure, which in turn allow governments to increase expenditure on welfare without eroding private consumption. Rose called this an era of 'treble affluence', because voters experience better social services, better take-home pay and better private consumption.[1] Electors are described as being altruistic during periods of economic prosperity because they feel secure in their employment and income and are therefore more likely to think of the 'other'.

By contrast, periods of retrenchment and economic stagnation are likely to lead to tensions between private and public consumption, with voters preferring to protect their private consumption even at the cost of eroding public consumption. The economic recessions of the early 1980s and 1990s have provided the opportunity for some governments to redefine the boundaries between public and private provision and also to experiment with different ways in delivering public services. Privatisation, the expansion of QUANGOs (quasi-autonomous non-government institutions) and quasi-markets represent attempts at redefining government. Equally reforms in pensions provision, unemployment costs and eligibility rules have all influenced voters' expectations of public provision.

The argument just outlined makes social policy something of an afterthought, an appendage to the economy; it follows that social policy has to correspond with the economic cycle. However, there is also the argument which points out that social policy cannot be separated from economic context. Social policy contributes directly to economic prosperity. According to this approach, social policy is perceived as having a major influence on issues of social solidarity and political stability and it creates the framework for stable macro-economic policy. Within the context of the welfare state, governments, employers and trades unions have been able to construct policies on pay and for dealing with inflation and investment. The welfare state has provided not only political legitimacy but also a process which allows for investment in health and education.

These have provided for a workforce which can respond to the challenges of flexibility and competitiveness.

The role of the state

The role of the state in relation to the economy is disputed. Six main positions might be identified, ranging from the least to the most interventionist.

The minimal state   The minimal state is a 'nightwatchman', in which the role of the state is limited. The main role of the state in relation to the economy is the setting of a framework including, for example, the legal basis of contract and the creation of units of exchange. The primary justification for this position is liberal: the state cannot legitimately intervene without jeopardising the freedom or rights of its citizens.

Subsidiarity   The second model is one in which the state is permitted to intervene, but intervention is subject to restraints in principle. The Catholic principle of subsidiarity argues for limitations of the actions of higher bodies like the state, and for priority to be given to decisions taken at the lowest possible levels of society – the individual, the family and the locality. A state can legitimately act to aid lesser social bodies. The combination of social responsibility with limitation on state activity has been a central tenet of Christian Democratic parties in Europe.

Pragmatic or functional intervention   A pragmatic approach to intervention judges the merits of intervention by the 'added value' it offers, and so to the extent to which it offers benefits in excess of costs, whether for individuals or for society as a whole. The German Sozialstaat, although strongly identified with the principle of subsidiarity, justifies intervention primarily on the basis of the benefits of social provision to the economy.

The mixed economy   Within the mixed economy, the state is itself involved in economic production, often in industries of national importance or in the provision of utilities which offer an infrastructure for industry. In relation to welfare, the most common forms of state activity relate to the provision of health care, education and pension provision, any of which might be administered through independent organisations or the market.

The managed economy   The Keynesian model offers the prospect of a managed economy, in which the state acts to plan, regulate and subsidise activity in order to maximise economic benefits to society. One of the implications of this is that the independence of the productive process is limited: intervention will take place to steer the direction of growth. This links the idea of the managed economy with a pattern of corporatism, where the state takes the main responsibility for planning but delegates activity to independent organisations. The managed economy can imply a minimal amount of direct intervention, and on that basis it could be seen as involving the state in less than a mixed economy. Much depends on the proportion of the economy which is affected by intervention, and in principle the managed economy affects every private enterprise.

Socialised production   The formerly communist states of eastern Europe claimed to be implementing a different kind of economic policy, in which production was controlled by the state and all citizens shared in the welfare of the society as members of a collective group. Lenin described the redistribution of income in terms of the division of a common social product, with parts being divided between wages, benefits and services and the activities of the state.

In Europe, the high levels of unemployment experienced in the last two decades have resulted in higher costs of social security programmes and in governments having to channel funds away from education and health to finance the social security budget. The process of privatisation and the introduction of quasi-markets in the delivery of core public services are now permanent features of the welfare state landscape. After the experiences of the 1980s it can no longer be assumed that government will become again involved in areas of public provision. While for over a century there has been a continuing expansion in state intervention, as we reach the beginning of the millennium the state is seeking to redefine itself.

Globalisation has also posed an important challenge to the role of the nation-state, because of the geographical limitations of a state's authority. In that context, some options seem more viable than others. The minimal state, pragmatism, and a mixed economy are all fully compatible with a complex, shifting pattern of production. Managing an economy or moving to strictly socialised production are much more difficult because of the limited control it is possible for a particular state to exercise. The principle of subsidiarity has another, interesting implication: that the level of intervention which is possible depends in part on the level at which activity is being undertaken. Where economic processes are supra-national, it may require a supra-national organisation to intervene. This is, of course, part of the justification for the formation of the European Union.

Public expenditure

The management of the economy is commonly judged in terms of the overall level of economic production which occurs. This is usually expressed in terms of the GNP (gross national product), or some variation of the idea, a figure which measures national income in the formal economy. The indicator is biased towards those engaged in economic activity and, in particular, to the upper reaches of the income distribution.[2] It is possible, in theory, for all the increase in national income to benefit the better-off and for this to be taken as an indication of a reduction in national poverty.

Governments manage a proportion of national income, and government expenditure is most usually expressed as a proportion of the GDP (gross domestic product – national income before trade). This is not the only criterion which is used; no less important is the issue of public sector deficits. The debate in the USA and France has been focused not so much on how much is spent as on how much is spent and not paid for. What the different approaches to public expenditure have in common is the view that government has to manage public expenditure within its income – a point which Keynesianism once disputed. This implies, in turn, that resources have to be allocated to different governmental functions, and spending on social welfare is commonly a major part of government expenditures. (It does not have to be, for two reasons. One is that it is perfectly possible to pay for social welfare in different ways, such as independent contributory funds, so that it does not appear on the government accounts. The second is that some countries do not count transfer payments – redistribution from one person to another – as expenditure at all.)

The allocation of resources at the level of government expenditure may be reflected in turn at lower levels. This is true, at least, of state-run welfare organisations, notably the National Health Service in the UK – a system which has been sufficiently successful in controlling costs to be imitated in southern European countries. But it is not true of systems which are distributed through market criteria (such as the provision of medical care in France or the Medicare system in the USA). Nor is it true of social security systems which are based on rights: what contributory pension funds have to pay out depends on the entitlements that people have earned and how long they live. These issues make the control of welfare expenditure difficult.

The dominant discourse in Europe in the 1990s accepts the linkage, however tenuous, between lack of competitiveness, unemployment and a welfare state which is acting as a burden on European economies. Unemployment in most European countries has in the 1990s reached peaks which had not been experienced at any time during the post-war period. Paradoxically, unemployment has not been of major concern for governments; the attempt to meet the criteria for monetary policy has been given priority. Governments have tended to argue that the problem of unemployment was structural, that the major concern should be to create frameworks for economic competitiveness, which in turn meant reducing the costs of social protection.

The welfare state after 1945 rested on the twin pillars of Keynesian economics and public finance through taxation and national insurance. The success in the financing of social policy depended on the assumptions on continued economic prosperity and low unemployment. The most effective way of controlling expenditure is to match income to expenditure. This, in general, implies that liabilities are limited while maximizing income. Liabilities can be limited by reducing entitlements – a process increasingly associated with greater selectivity. (Andries notes that, despite preconceptions to the contrary, it is the universal benefits which have been most vulnerable to cuts, and selective benefits which have proved most robust.[3]) But they can be limited much more effectively if people are put in the position where they do not need to claim – by ensuring that, wherever possible, they are fully engaged in economic activity. Income, similarly, is maximized when people are earning and paying tax or contributions, and reduced when they are not.

Integrating the excluded

A crucial aspect of the control of expenditure is policy to minimise economic marginality and exclusion. Exclusion is one of the principal issues which arises in the discussion of the changing economy. Economic exclusion is not simply equivalent to being in work, because some of those who are in work are economically marginal – in low-paid, temporary and precarious work. Nor is it quite the same as people who are not economically active, because many people who are not economically active – particularly pensioners – may still be covered by solidaristic networks which offer social protection. A range of people may effectively be excluded because they are not part of the labour market: they include single parents with childcare responsibilities, people with chronic sickness and physical disability, and people with obsolete skills forced into early retirement. As a shorthand, it is possible to focus on the problems of unemployment and precarious employment.

The main possibility of integrating those who are excluded lies within economic policy. For macro-economists, unemployment is principally a function of the level of economic activity. Keynesian economists, by contrast, see the role of government expenditure in very different terms; the constructive use of expenditure can be used to stimulate production, either through increasing aggregate demand or through selective stimulation of chosen areas of production. Liberal macro-economists put their emphasis on minimising the arbitrary nature of government in the conduct of economic policy. The nature of economic policy in a liberal environment should be conducted according to constitutional rules, which means that government makes explicit its intentions on economic policy. This means that government expenditure should be financed through taxation rather than relying on borrowing so that voters receive a clear message of their opportunity costs between increased public services and less personal consumption.

Liberal micro-economists, by contrast, are concerned with the presence of rigidities in the labour market. These obstacles include institutional factors, social considerations and the effect of collective action on the labour market. Micro-economists would argue that each of these set of factors is likely to influence the supply or demand side of the labour market. The flexibility of the labour market depends on the movement in prices to reflect changes in the demand and supply of labour. Interventions by government on rights against dismissal, national insurance, personal taxation and minimum wages are all likely to increase the cost of labour, which means that either employers would demand less labour because of the higher costs or fewer workers would make themselves available for work because of the low price. The conduct of government should therefore be to create competitive labour markets where there is equal access for suppliers and consumers. According to labour market economists, therefore, government can reform the labour market in four critical ways:

1 reducing the duration of job search by reducing the rates of social security payments;
2 increasing labour supply by reducing personal taxation rates;
3 reforming trade union immunities so that the supply side of the trade unions becomes more responsive to changes in price;
4 removing minimum wage legislation, since this is likely to increase the price of labour on the employer, thus resulting in an actual fall in the demand for labour.

If the Keynesian view is correct, some of these measures would be counter-productive: reducing social security payments and minimum wages will reduce the aggregate level of demand, and so reduce the demand for production and employment. Equally, reducing workers' rights and diminishing union membership might be seen as a way of exacerbating the problems of marginality and exclusion which labour market policy is seeking to address.

However, European governments have now firmly abandoned fiscal policy as the means for reducing unemployment. The Keynesian approach to demand management has been displaced by the argument of supply-side economics, of reducing labour costs as a way of increasing demand for labour. One of the main routes through which the problems of unemployment and sub-employment have been addressed is through job creation and training. There is a significant difference between the two: training depends on the assumption that work will be available for those who acquire the skills, job creation that it will not. An interesting fusion has been developed in the French system, where claimants of the basic income support benefit, the *Revenu Minimum d'Insertion*, are required to negotiate a 'Contract of Insertion' with a social worker. The contract of insertion can be based in employment, or in other aspects of social integration; the responsible body, the

Commission Locale d'Insertion, also has the responsibility to negotiate with local agencies and enterprises to provide a sufficient number
of opportunities to make the contract meaningful. The emphasis has
fallen on the excluded person, rather than the economy: policies
which formerly were treated as part of the management of a national
economy have become focused on individual casework.

The economics of postmodernity

In the postmodern economy, the structures and processes of economic production and consumption become fluid and uncertain.
Concepts such as markets, competitiveness and flexible labour
markets are not value-free; they represent contestable sites. Flexibility at one level means creating a framework which enables
employees to lower their wages so that their business remains competitive in the context of the globalised economy. Flexibility could
also mean investment in human capital, that is, on expenditure in
education and training so that employees can meet the challenges
of competitiveness through higher skills and the ability to produce
goods at a level of higher added value. Flexibility can therefore be
correlated with reducing social protection costs because these are
seen as a burden to the employer, but flexibility could also mean
increasing social protection costs as means of investing in human
capital.

The break with standardisation of full employment and full-time
work has given way to pluralised forms of working, including part-
time employment which usually is correlated with low pay and
casualisation. The job for life is replaced by flexible jobs and fragmented work which, in turn, result in under-employment and unemployment. Economic growth is no longer likely to achieve full
employment.

> Economic upturns no longer signal the end of unemployment.
> 'Rationalizing' now means cutting not creating jobs, and tech-
> nological and managerial progress is measured by 'slimming
> down' the work force. . . . Jobs for life are no more. As a
> matter of fact jobs as such, as we once understood them, are
> no more. Without them there is little room for life lived as a
> project, for long-term planning and far-reaching hopes. Be
> grateful for the bread you eat today and do not think too far
> ahead. The symbol of wisdom is no longer the savings book;

it is now, at least for those able to afford them, being wise, the credit cards and a walletful of them.[4]

The shift in macro-economic thinking from a Keynesian to a market approach has meant that governments have abandoned the concept of creating employment through fiscal policy. Instead, the emphasis is on supply-side economics and the economics of flexible labour markets. Supply-side economics puts on the focus on reducing costs to the employers, moderating wage demands, reducing the influence of trade unions in wage bargaining, and reducing social costs. Labour market reforms therefore create a climate of contracts between the employers and the individualised worker. The attempts to regulate wages, restate workers' rights in the workplace and bargain around social rights are seen as interventions in the workings of the labour markets and therefore a hindrance to employment.

Beck's argument has been that the dual dynamics of globalisation and increased individualisation require a break with conventional policies.[5] The globalised economy makes transparent the limits of the nation-state. Governments in the 1990s are more ready to admit their limited autonomy in the management of national economies and are also more likely to utilise the concept of the global economy in seeking to reform and restructure national economies. Beck contrasts the duality of globalisation and individualisation with the concepts of collectivism and the nation-state and argues that welfare states need to be contextualised within the duality of collectivisim and the nation-state and that therefore the new challenges of globalisation and individualisation seek to redefine the relevance of welfare state. The globalised economy has contributed to the decline in the influence of the nation-state and therefore national governments in the 1990s are less able to deal with the risks of the globalised economy, including economic, social and environmental risks. Increasingly, the language of competitiveness and more flexible labour markets translates itself as a series of policies of retrenchment in the context of social policy. Social policy becomes equated with social costs and therefore perceived to be a burden on competitiveness and employment. Reducing social costs usually means reducing pension liabilities, health costs and social security costs.

The welfare state was born out of a sense of collective responsibility, but patterns of universalism and equality have given way to individualism. Ironically, the welfare state itself has contributed to the dissolving of class, gender and family and has moved collective biographies to individualised biographies where, increasingly, individuals are encouraged to think that they are involved in making choices within a 'capitalist' economy. Whilst analysis of class might still be appropriate as a form of understanding inequality, collective identities have dissolved. The tendency to differentiation of life styles has been made possible by consumer society, which tends to emphasise identity in terms of consumer goods. People with the same income level persist in leading different life styles – there is no shared community of experience. Class position no longer predicts a person's outlook; the individual is removed from traditional ties to ties within the labour market and as a consumer. Labour market risks become individualised experiences.

Part of the process has been a change in the nature of welfare itself. The rights which people have, their social situation, and the relationships they take part in, are particular, individualised and distinctive, rather than universal and general. This does not necessarily mean a reduced commitment to public expenditure: Maurice Mullard's analyses of public expenditure accounts in the UK have tended to show that the reductions made in public expenditure have been marginal, and mainly focused on capital expenditure, holding down public sector pay and reducing expenditure on defence.[6] But a concern with public expenditure alone conceals a revolution in expectations and patterns of provision: it is the relative role of the state in social protection which has reduced, with an increased reliance on benefits from a range of sources and a growing complexity in the systems which provide them.

The kind of economy which is represented in the analysis of postmodern society is also profoundly unequal. Difference for some is disadvantage for others; flexibility can mean precariousness. The new economic order can be empowering, and for many it is integrative, but it is also often exclusive, restrictive and unequal. This prompts two areas of concern. The first, considered in the next chapter, is with the political framework and with the scope of democracy to empower citizens. The second, considered in the final chapter, is to examine the scope for social justice.

Chapter 14

The political framework

Democracy and welfare

The changes in the political framework of developed countries in the period since the Second World War are suggestive of a degree of convergence, often through conscious imitation of 'successful' countries. There has been a trend for western-style 'democracy' to become established in a range of countries, including many in which the application of democratic principles seems rather fragile. The key elements of democracy in this sense are a combination of government accountable to an electorate, the supremacy of the law, and the protection of the rights of individuals and minorities. The existence of democratic institutions is not enough to explain what kind of welfare system might be introduced. The key distinctions between different kinds of welfare state – like the coverage of the system, the commitment to redistribution, or the extent of commodification and reliance on the market – are not predicated by the political system. On that basis, a concern with political processes or institutions may seem marginal to a concern with social policy.

The trend to democratization does, however, have important implications for the development of welfare, both negative and positive. In negative terms, the states of the former Eastern Europe have abandoned principles of basic security and universalism along with the ideology of comprehensive state intervention. In positive terms, democracy has been associated not only with economic development, but with the protection of the rights of the poor. Famine, Drèze and Sen argue, is produced in poor countries not by shortage of food, but by lack of entitlement; people die of hunger because they are not entitled to eat the food which exists. The starvation suffered by millions in both the Irish famine of the mid-nineteenth century or the Chinese famine of the 1950s was caused not by lack of available food but by the failure to make it available to those who could not afford to buy or transport it.

> Famine is, by its very nature, a social phenomenon (it involves the inability of large groups of people to establish command over food in the society in which they live) . . . it has to be recognised that even when the prime mover in a famine is a natural occurrence such as a flood or a drought, what its impact will be on the population will depend on how society is organised.[1]

A famine has never occurred in a democratic state. It is not completely clear why this should be the case – it is probably true that democratic states tend to be richer, and there is a temptation to say that states where famine occurs were obviously not democratic enough – but the observation alone constitutes a very powerful argument for democratic government.

The meaning of democracy

Accounts of democracy can be located within two major perspectives. These are liberal democracy and communitarian democracy. Each of these models is concerned with a series of core assumptions which makes the models distinct. Advocates for liberal democracy emphasise the ethics of negative freedom and the need to protect the individual from the coercive powers of the state; communitarian democracy seeks to emphasise positive freedom and the potential for increasing the rights of the individual through the community. At another level, the divisions between liberalism and communitarian democracy might be taken to represent an argument between representative and participative models of democracy.

Each of these perspectives is complex; each contains different schools of thought. They seem to be incommensurate, because in each case the 'story' they tell seeks to provide a competing interpretation of what should be the concerns of modern democracy.

Liberal democracy

The idea of liberal democracy was mentioned briefly in Chapter 6 in the discussion of social democracy. There are many different interpretations, however, and if we want to understand the nature of debates about democracy a more thorough consideration is needed. Although the advocates of liberal democracy are agreed about the central position of the individual, there are differences between those liberals who argue for an ultra-minimalist state, as articulated in the work of Hayek and Nozick, and those liberals who seek a more pragmatic and interventionist liberal state which can enhance the rights and opportunities for the individual, as suggested by Rorty, Rawls and Brittan.

The ultra minimalist view of liberal democracy   The ultra-minimalist view of liberal democracy establishes individual rights as essential to the doctrine of liberal democracy. Individual liberty is seen as the emancipation of the subject, who was historically treated by the monarch as a body to be disposed of without any forms of recall to the law or justice. Individual rights are inalienable and non-negotiable. The individual has to be perceived as a rational agent capable of making decisions, which are of equal value to decisions made by other individuals. Individuals have to be treated with respect and dignity as ends in themselves: 'individuals are ends and not merely means; they may not be sacrificed or used for the achieving of other ends without their consent.'[2]

Establishing rights within a democracy is essential because it confirms our rights to separate existences for individuals: to have the rights to visions of personal life projects, which are not dependent on others. The political process is to be treated with suspicion and caution, because it is more fickle and unjust than the market place. Inequalities which emerge within the marketplace are just, because individuals meet as sovereign individuals; in contrast, inequalities which result from resource allocation by the political process are unjust because these inequalities relate to inequalities of access to the political process. Those likely to benefit through the political process are the political elite and those who have the knowledge and access to the political process.

Pragmatic liberalism   In contrast to the libertarian vision of inalienable rights, the pragmatist defence of liberal democracy rests on the assumption that the potential of democracy is limited and that individuals should not have expectations which democracy cannot deliver. However, pragmatists also accept that democracy will continue to be a potential for political choice where political parties will continue to compete for people's votes. The pragmatic tradition is anti-foundational, which means that pragmatists favour a world of universal doubts – a suspicion of those who appear to have ready-made explanations. Pragmatists are therefore suspicious of the advocates of Libertarian and Communitarian democracy, and of the argument that creating a more democratic culture is likely to lead to greater tolerance. There is no craving for absolutes, but rather a concern for knowledge which is likely to be tentative, open to interpretation and always subject to correction. The pragmatist defends liberal democracy because it provides a context for compromise and negotiation. The threats to liberal democracy are posed by those who have fanatical visions for society and who have no tolerance for the visions of others. Liberal democracy is therefore threatened by those who take advantage of liberal institutions to pursue doctrine and use democracy as a means to an end rather than defending democracy as an end in itself. Pragmatists accept the precariousness of liberal democracy. Within this framework pragmatists accept that the world is made of pluralities but that these pluralities have to be bounded within a context of liberal democracy.

> The type of pluralism that represents what is best in our pragmatic tradition is an engaged fallibilistic pluralism. Such a pluralistic ethos places new responsibilities upon each of us. For it means taking our fallibility seriously – resolving that however much we are committed to our styles of thinking we are willing to listen to others without denying or suppressing the otherness of the other.[3]

The question of whether liberal democracy has failed rests on a conflation of arguments on democracy. The concept of democracy represents an admixture of normative arguments as to what democracy ought to be and which tend to live alongside the pragmatic arguments of how democracy seems to work in modern societies. Bobbio, for example, has argued that the future of liberal democracy depends on lowering our normative expectations of democracy and constructing some 'minimal' expectations of those who continue to adhere to democratic principles.[4] He therefore urges that a minimal democracy should be characterised by a set of rules concerning who is eligible to vote, the rights of political parties, and free and frequent elections: a set of rules which establish who is authorised to rule and which procedures to be applied. Yet democracy needs to offer real alternatives since politics is about conflicts of what needs to done, whilst at the same time it needs to give priority to liberal rights.

Bobbio seems to argue that criticisms of modern democracy rest on what he calls the Six Broken Promises of Democracy. These are:

1   The persistence of pluralism and politics as practised through interest groups. This form of politics generates and maintains inequality, and pluralism is identified with those who organise themselves and gain access to political goods at the cost of those who are on the outside and remain marginalised.

2   Political parties are mainly concerned with becoming and remaining the incumbent government. Their main concern is therefore to produce policies desirable to electoral majorities. According to Heller, electoral majorities tend to thread together a form of political consensus which is often oppressive to those who are on the outside of that consensus.[5] Electoral majorities reflect a defence of the status quo.

3   The survival of oligarchy – representative democracy generates new forms of political elites rather than a process of participation.

4   Limited spaces for democracy, the process of democracy through the bureaucracy of political parties sets limits to the political agenda. The classical vision of democracy is corrupted by the more pragmatic arguments that democracy is a method of choosing between competing elites.

5   Invisible power is what Hannah Arendt describes as the 'rule by nobody'. The influence and impact of the welfare state and the bureaucracy of government reduce the importance of the 'elected' assembly.

6   Democracy lives alongside the 'uneducated citizen' – modern democracy has been further corrupted because it seems to encourage passivity by the public, so that the political stage is left to the few while the majority becomes the silent audience. Modern democracy is limited to electoral process whilst other forms of participation are discouraged.

Communitarian democracy: the participatory model of democracy

The participatory model emphasises the normative element of democracy and therefore seeks to ask how democracies ought to work. The model is characterised by an attempt to provide an agenda for democracy, for providing opportunities for participation but also pointing out that participation should not be left to narrow aspects of electoral democracy.

> The problem of building a democratic society is thus one of a dynamic interaction of rules and actors with the actors rendering the rules more democratic, and the increasingly democratic rules rendering the actors more firmly committed to and skilled in democratic participation and decision making. We term this process a democratic dynamic.[6]

The communitarians point to the limits of liberal democratic principles, arguing that individuals cannot be perceived to exist in a vacuum or as unencumbered selves. Individuals are an inherent part of their community and it is within communities that ethics of democracy and citizenship are created. It is communities which create opportunities and public spaces, that can then generate options which guaranteeing diversity and pluralities of views and therefore a more discursive model of democracy. Freedom of the individual cannot be perceived in a void but can only be understood within the wider social context – it is the community which therefore defines freedom. Communitarian democracy is intended to allow for the articulation of a plurality of demands and interests. Freedom and democracy do not depend on definitions agreed *a priori*; democracy and freedom continue to derive their meanings within specific social contexts.

According to this approach it is not sufficient to understand how democracy works at present; it is necessary to establish a culture of democracy. The ethics of participation in decision making should not be confined to the electoral process but also to other aspects of our daily lives. This means the right to participate at our place of work, that is, to be involved in decisions on investment which are likely to affect our daily lives. It also entails economic democracy and establishing consumer rights against monopoly suppliers. Finally, there is social democracy and the recognition that at present democracy is confined to the public sphere, which mitigates against increased participation by women but also limits the boundaries between what is perceived to be the public as opposed to the private sphere.

The vision of participatory democracy seeks to encourage a public culture where the process of participation is likely to result in a more and better informed citizen. This vision seeks to revitalise the Greek classic of the polis, where it was argued that the primary objective of a society was to denaturalise the individual. The natural human being in this context led a privatised life. The process of democracy sought to turn the individual into a public citizen.

> [The individual] loses his personal identity and becomes a part of a purposive social unit. Here the group absorbs all his resources, emotional as well as physical. And this is the very essence of the psychological transformation of man into a citizen.[7]

However, whilst there might be some general agreement as to the meaning of participatory democracy, there are two major variants within this model which need to be investigated further. For example, there is a tension between those who argue for substantive democracy but still seek to preserve the homogeneity of community, in contrast to those who argue for a more heterogeneous approach to democracy and who seek to constitute community rather than assume that community actually exists. The concept of a community which is perceived to be homogenous has been criticised for being exclusive; community has been also criticised for being dominated by patriarchy and also racism.

Communitarian democracy: radical democracy

The most complete statement for a radical democracy has come from the Budapest school. Their central argument is that the aim of radical democracy should be to complete the agenda of procedural democracy:

1   positive elimination of property – rather than nationalising property as an aim to create a more equal society;
2   the expansion of participation in industry and the workplace giving employees the rights of shareholders;

3   equal recognition of need – to recognise that needs are diverse
     and plural and that radical democracy cannot promise to pro-
     duce abundance to meet all needs;
4   the creation of a new public sphere to allow equal recognition of
     all needs, encouraging public debate, collective social con-
     science, and a power structure that contributes to compromise
     so that no group feels maltreated or rolled over by majority
     views.

The central ethics of a radical democracy are the recognition that
tensions and conflicts will not be eliminated. Individual liberty, the
pursuit of equality and democracy are given equal value. The
moral maxims allow for the freedom of the individual, justice and
an end to suffering. These maxims are not too much to expect of
individuals – they do not interfere with individual freedom; they
aim to stop exploitation and unnecessary suffering.[8] The new radical
democracy does not ask for complete altruism, for individuals to
surrender self-interest but, rather, that people become less myopic
and instead show a greater understanding of how their actions
affect others.

   The Budapest School recognises two interpretations of socialism:
one is the socialism that is committed to equality in decision making;
the second is that socialism is the negation of capitalism. According
to the Budapest School, the latter does not guarantee more freedom
or more equality. Instead it is now equated with bureaucracy,
injustice and inefficiency.

> There cannot be more freedom than the right and the possibility
> of equal participation in decision-making processes in terms of
> the democratic concept of freedom. In terms of the democratic
> concept of freedom, the more everyone has the right and the
> possibility to participate the freer people are. Liberation can
> thus be conceived as a lengthy process in which everyone has
> the right and the very increasing possibility for participating.
> And that is what democratic freedom is about.[9]

Pluralist democracy: the discourse model of democracy

In contrast to the vision of radical democracy, there is the view that
the central concern of democracy should be the project that defends
pluralism. It suggests that there are forms of oppression beside class

oppression, such as oppressions related to gender, race, disability and other forms of disadvantage. These oppressions cannot be reduced to class or to other explanations which depend on other reductionist theories. It is an approach which accepts the concept of agency where individuals are neither always victims or agents of oppression but that resources for oppression take different forms. Within this context it is therefore the realisation that people have a diversity of needs, that their potentials and abilities are hindered by factors which are not economic. Once these axioms are accepted then wider implications can be derived. First, there is the implication that the interests of the working class and of production are not dominant within the project substantive democracy. Second, this perspective denies the presence and the emergence of one emancipatory category where neither the working class nor the women's movement are likely to be the single categories of emancipation. Instead, emancipation has to be individualistic without a predetermined view of the good society.

The project of pluralist democracy recognises diversity, conflicts of interests and priorities but also recognises the common aim of replacing oppression. The programme of pluralist democracy starts with the assumption that differences are to be celebrated. The recognition of these differences is likely to lead to alliances and coalitions which are founded on the recognition of difference. New social movements therefore are likely to succeed because of respect and toleration of diversity rather than the false attempt to construct a homogeneous programme. In contrast to radical democracy, the programme of cultural democracy does not limit its claims to increased participation but rather to broader issues of the rights of the individual, the recognition of diversity of interests and the view that emancipation is more than the right to participate in decision making.

It would seem that the pragmatist wants a greater emphasis on the natural and private world where the version of democracy is similar to that developed by Barber, which the author called 'Thin Democracy'.[10] The adherence to thin democracy is founded on the premise of individualism where democratic values correspond with the values of self-interest. Thin democracy is described by Barber as being precarious and provisional because the commitment to democracy is limited to the pursuit of self-interest. The voter pursuing self-interest may therefore abandon democracy for other forms of politics if other political systems seem to offer something better. It is not sufficient to be narrow democrats where commitment is limited to self-interest; there has to be a commitment to participation and a positive definition of liberty. The pragmatist tradition also embraces a negative framework to liberty in the sense that it points only to the negative nature of the state, the arbitrary nature of politics, 'the burden of public expenditure and coercive taxation'.

The adherents of thin democracy point to the duality of enlightened self-interest and the cynical nature of the political process. The political process is more akin to a zoo of cunning foxes and lions, of animals which prey upon the unsuspecting individual who only makes the demand to be left alone by the state. To escape the political jungle, market liberals urge for limits to be put on government through a written constitution, freedom of information and a bill of rights. Market liberals therefore emphasise the need to construct civil society as the alternative to the public/political society.

This vision of democracy needs to be contrasted to Hannah Arendt's vision that the major contribution to progress has been the endeavour to establish an artificial world – where artificial means the setting of public institutions and political processes which encourage the ethics of public participation and public argument. Arendt compared the artificial world to the natural world of the family and employment. The natural world is easier to deal with because the responsibilities are easier to discern; the individual takes fewer risks – there is no need to negotiate or compromise with others in engaging in the artificial world.[11] Democracy is an artefact – made by humans – and in its nature it remains a continuing project. Democracy continues to be an ideal. It is as yet not in place and therefore cannot be empirically researched. Arblaster states: 'Democracies exist because we have invented them, because they are in our minds and insofar as we grasp how to keep them well and alive.'[12]

According to Arblaster, the main task of democrats is not to defend democracy but to create democracy.[13] Democracy asks for continuing vigilance. Democracy represents a continuing tension between the 'ought' – the continuing project of political striving – and the 'is' of democracy – which tends to set the limits and constraints on the project. All discussions on democracy seem to revolve around three issues: popular sovereignty, equality and self-government.[14] Popular sovereignty represents the attempt to construct the sovereign individual where all individuals are unequal and, because they are unequal, they are interdependent – hence the need for equal sovereignty. Furthermore, sovereignty for the individual also means that the rights of the individual are not to be negotiated away. No majority has the right to erode the rights of minorities.

Arguing that democracy is 'power of the people' represents a word-for-word definition, yet democracy is more than a group of words. Democracy stands for something and it is therefore not sufficient to look at the literal meaning of democracy but, more important, that we understand that democracy seeks to combine the is and the ought. Democracy is therefore both a descriptive and a normative concept. In this sense we cannot empirically test for democracy – the empirical approach only captures the micro meaning of democracy whilst democracy itself has much more of a macro meaning. According to Sartori:

> To avoid starting out on the wrong foot we must keep in mind, then, that (a) the democratic ideal does not define the democratic reality and, vice versa, a real democracy is not, and cannot be, the same as an ideal one, and that (b) democracy results from, and is shaped by, the interactions between its ideals and its reality, the pull of an ought and the resistance of an is.[15]

A system of democracy must provide opportunities and sites which generate options, diversity and pluralities of views and therefore more freedom. Democracy has to be perceived to be an ongoing project to lower and reduce the arbitrary nature of decision making within public institutions. This means that democracy needs to be constantly created – supporters of democracy have to defend democracy. The process of democracy can be associated with limiting the powers of others and therefore increasing our freedom. Within a democratic context we are less likely to be coerced to do certain things or think in certain ways. Democracy also facilitates a sphere of opposition, a system which allows for the articulation of a plurality of demands and interests and it is the ability to recognise differences that increases personal freedom.

Developing entitlements

Rights

Rights have to be understood at several levels. Some rights are moral, based in social norms (or, some would argue, universal codes of behaviour); some are legal, and legal rights may or may not have a moral basis. The main test of legal rights is that they have some kind of sanction, and so they can be enforced. The term 'welfare rights' is mainly used to refer to legal rights for people. On the face of the matter, moral rights which lack any means of enforcement are of limited relevance to welfare, but there are three important arguments to the contrary. The first is that moral issues matter in the world of politics. Policies are made, and laws are passed, because of social norms. Second, statements of rights are important. Where moral rights have been affirmed – for example, in the Universal Declaration of Human Rights, or the UN Declaration of the Rights of the Child – they may still have a persuasive effect. Third, a legal right, like a right to rehousing, may be worth little in a society which disregards it or fails to protect vulnerable people; a moral right, like the right to health, may carry more weight even though it is virtually unenforceable. In cases where legal rights exist which are not approved morally, there may be profound problems in enforcing the right. The term 'stigma' has been used to refer to the position in which people are reluctant to claim benefits or services to which they are entitled.[16] Although the scope and effects of stigma are disputed, there are certainly general problems of low utilisation and limited access which become aggravated in relation to the poorest claimants.

A second important distinction lies between particular and general rights. People have a particular right if someone has undertaken a personal obligation towards them (for example, as the result of a promise, a contract, or an injurious action); they have a general right if it applies to everyone else in similar circumstances (for example, as children, old people, or mentally ill people). The rights which people gain in the market are usually particular; the rights people gain from politics are usually general. Particular rights have been especially important in the development of social welfare in some European countries. The strategy followed in French social policy, which has been influential in Europe, has been to build on solidaristic social networks, progressively extending the scope of solidarity to include those who previously were excluded. The original basis of these networks was a combination of preexisting solidarities, like the solidarities of family and community, with contractual rights gained through the development of mutual aid. In the same way, arguments about rights in developing countries have relied on economic development, and progressive integration of people into the network of relationships built on the formal economy, as the primary route through which entitlements can be established.

A third issue which ought to be considered is whether rights are individual or collective. Although most discussions of rights are based on the position of individuals, arguments have been made for a different emphasis, establishing rights for disadvantaged groups or peoples.[17] This is a complex subject, but one which has been scarcely examined because of the absence of appropriate mechanisms in many legal systems for redressing the situation of groups. (The main exception is found in the USA – not the existence of 'class actions', because class actions are still taken by and on behalf of identifiable individuals, but rather the Brandeis brief, which allows consideration of the consequences to a wider society of the actions under review.) A focus on the group or community may be especially appropriate and enforceable in circumstances where rights are enshrined in the obligations of states towards their citizens.

Citizenship

Within the democratic tradition, the primary defence of rights has been expressed in terms of citizenship. Citizenship is a basic status, which gives each person who holds it the ability to be recognised in a political community. It has been described as the 'right to have rights'. In feudal times, people were not citizens: they did not have political rights but rather were the property of their lords. The modern idea of citizenship has its roots in the Enlightenment, the intellectual movement of the seventeenth and eighteenth centuries which sought to substitute the language of reason and rights for tradition and divine authority. The language of rights associated with citizenship was also central to the Enlightenment since the latter represented a struggle against ideology, a means of unmasking and making the world more transparent through the process of free dialogue and the acceptance of the better argument.

The model of citizenship which has emerged subsequently is more complex. The Marshallian view of citizenship, considered in Chapter 6 on social democracy, extended the idea to cover social rights in an inclusive and universalist framework. The dominant models of rights and citizenship have been, for most of this century, founded in concepts of individual right, universality and membership of a political community. There are contradictions within these concepts – it has been difficult, for example, to argue both that individuals have general rights as human beings and that their rights must be framed in terms of membership of a specific political community. But the concepts are also being stretched. They are no longer solely individual, general and based in the nation-state; they are just as likely to be collective and particular. One of the implications of a global economy is the development of cross-national patterns of solidarity founded in particular rights.

This does not simply resolve the difficulties inherent in framing welfare rights; rather, it presents new problems and challenges. The development of citizenship as a social status has a huge potential for exclusion. Particular rights encourage diversity and difference; they can also legitimate inequality. Collective and group rights help to redefine citizenship, but they can also put individuals in other groups at a disadvantage. In these circumstances, it is important to see these rights not simply in terms of the material advantages they convey but in a political context – understanding how the political framework can be used to empower people and redress disadvantage.

The welfare state

There is no simply agreed concept of the welfare state. The term refers variously to the delivery of social services by the state; the strategy of developing interrelated social services to deal with a wide range of social problems; or an ideal in which services are provided comprehensively and at the best level possible. Asa Briggs identifies three directions of movement:

- a guarantee of minimum incomes to individuals and families irrespective of the market value of their work or property;
- the reduction of insecurity by protecting individuals and families against income loss crisis contingencies; and

- ensuring that all citizens, without distinction of class or status, are offered the best standards available in a range of social services.[18]

The power of the idea of the welfare state has perhaps faded in recent years. In part, it reflects disillusionment with the role of the nation-state, which has been condemned both from the right (by liberals) and from the left (by neo-Marxists). In part, it reflects an under-standing of the nature of welfare, which relies not so much on the formal mechanisms of social services as on the relationships which exist in a society. It might also be seen as a recognition that different kinds of welfare regimes – like the development of particular rights linked to employment in formal economies – may have served the population better than a system which seemed to rest in donative rights, rights which were given by the government rather than estab-lished through social solidarity. Titmuss condemned the idea of the welfare state because it induced complacency, and because it stood in the way of a broader internationalist perspective.

There is a sense, though, in which any democratic country becomes a welfare state. Government, Edmund Burke once wrote, is a contrivance of human wisdom to provide for human wants. If a state is at all responsive to the needs and wishes of its citizens, it will provide or ensure the provision of basic social protection, protecting them against the consequences of social insecurity. That, perhaps, is why democracies do not have famines.

Chapter 15

Social welfare and social justice

Social justice: towards a just society

The word 'justice' has many meanings, but it is also used in two primary senses. For some, 'just' action is whatever is good, right, or desirable, which is how Plato used the term.[1] Although the term is little used in this way in ordinary language, writers frequently confuse issues of justice with other questions of morality – John Rawls, for example, makes liberty an integral principle.[2] The problem with adding principles on to just action is that it ends up meaning nothing more than 'morally approved'. This is not completely meaningless, because it does represent an important principle: that the way things are in society is not necessarily the way they have to be, and that moral principles are relevant to the way society is organised. This stands in opposition to the kind of individualistic argument made by Hayek and the New Right. What it does not do, unfortunately, is to explain what action should be taken. In the UK, the Labour Party's Commission on Social Justice ended up with a programme so wide that it seemed to have lost any sense of purpose – effectively writing a party manifesto rather than a document on justice.[3]

The second sense of justice concerns justice as fairness, which is how it was taken by Aristotle.[4] An action is 'fair' if it treats people proportionately to certain agreed criteria: for Aristotle, 'the just is the proportionate'. Social justice is basically a distributive principle: it concerns the proportions in which people should contribute to and receive things from society. The criteria which have been proposed as the basis for distribution are complex: they have included human rights, need, desert, contribution to society and hereditary status, among many others. Defining appropriate criteria is essential to any conception of social justice. A distribution based on need tends to be much more egalitarian than one based on desert; distribution according to human rights, or the rights of citizenship, may be more equal than either.

What is just is not, on this account, simply the same as what is 'good' or 'right'. An action is good when beneficial consequences are produced or intended (there are many complexities here, but they are not central to the argument). An action is right when it is morally approved or desired; justice is often right, because it is approved in itself, but it may not be when it conflicts with other principles like liberty and democracy.

Social justice is not necessarily egalitarian. A principle of proportionate distribution can legitimate disadvantage: for example, in cases where distribution is proportionate to contribution to society, the consequences may be very unequal. However, justice does presume equality in circumstances where there are no relevant distinguishing criteria – because the due proportions cannot be distinguished. This implies that, in any principle of distributive justice, differences must be justified.

What would make society more just? Clearly, part of the answer is a greater degree of equality, because inequalities have to be justified; but it is only part, because a principle of justice can in some circumstances argue for some degree of inequality. The effect of compensation for disability, recognition of service to the community, or protection through insurance can all have inegalitarian consequences, but they are widely recognised as legitimate principles. They do not justify the gross inequalities which come from inherited wealth, accidents of fortune or even intelligent manipulation of market opportunities – inequalities justified by Nozick in terms of legitimate succession of property rights.[5] Social justice is based on a moral assessment of distributive consequences. Hayek argues that morality is irrelevant to distributive consequences,[6] but that is not a widely held view: many of the advocates of distribution through the market (like de Jouvenel or Acton[7]) try to justify it in moral terms. This is not really susceptible to argument: either one considers that the distribution of resources is subject to moral judgment, or one does not.

Contractarianism

In *A Theory of Justice*, Rawls argued that a just society would seek to balance the question of redistribution with the liberty of the individual. Rawls' concept of justice is based on an imagined 'contract', in which people are asked to decide what a fair apportionment of resources would be, without knowing in advance what the consequences would be for themselves personally. In Rawls' terms, the contract is formed under a 'veil of ignorance'. Within a contractual framework, Rawls argues that it is possible to construct a constitution which ensures that all individuals are treated as equals, where there is freedom of conscience, freedom of thought and freedom of speech but, also, under that veil of ignorance or original position, these individuals will also construct a theory of just entitlement. Although agreement can be reached to construct the constitution which protects the rights of all individuals, the question of entitlements will not lead to similar agreements.[8]

The model of justice this favours is Platonic rather than Aristotelian; justice consists of what people find acceptable rather than what is proportionate. Rawls's view is that it is possible to put the rights of the individual and questions concerning the distribution of resources in a lexical order. The first step is to take the rights of the individual as inalienable and non-negotiable; from there it is possible to go on to construct a theory of justice which takes into consideration economic and social issues.

Rawls begins from the proposition that in a just society, inequalities need to be justified. He points to two problems associated with inequality. The first is that inequality in basic liberties amounts to a denial of liberty. The second is that inequality of opportunity produces undesirable social consequences, because it fails to make use of human resources. A distribution is efficient if no one can be made better off without making someone else worse off; inefficiency implies that people are worse off than they need to be. If the distribution of income acts as barrier to entry for certain individuals so that these individuals, because of lack of income, cannot explore fully their abilities, then resources are not being allocated efficiently. From this, he establishes two main principles:

> The first principle of equal liberty is the primary standard for the constitutional convention. Its main requirements are that the fundamental liberties of the person and liberty of conscience

and freedom of thought be protected . . . The second principle dictates that social and economic policies be aimed at maximising the long-term expectations of the least advantaged under conditions of fair equality of opportunity.[9]

The main way in which inequalities of income or status can be justified are that such inequalities would be acceptable. According to Rawls, inequality can be justified if it can be proved that inequality is likely to benefit everyone, including those on the lowest incomes. If high income differentials do provide incentives for high income earners to generate economic prosperity which benefits the poor then Rawls argues that income inequality can be justified. This argument is similar to the 'trickle-down theory' in economics which suggests that higher income generates economic activity which helps everyone in a society. He calls this the 'difference principle'.

Rawls disaggregates the question of just entitlement under two criteria: those of equal opportunity and access. Equal opportunity is necessary because if income or status act as a barrier to entry to offices and certain positions, then inequality is likely to generate inefficiency because of the monopoly power of income concentration but also because income inequality is likely to deny liberty. On the second criterion, that the distribution of income should be to everyone's benefit, Rawls argues that individuals might decide on the difference principle and thus justify income inequality as long as that rule benefits everyone. This position has been criticised: it ignores issues of social class,[10] and the problems of exclusion associated with inequality.

Equality and redistribution

Because differences have to be justified, justice tends to imply equality. Egalitarian policies are commonly framed in three ways. There is the prevention of disadvantage in access to services or to equal treatment. There is the removal of disadvantage in competition with others, which is equality of opportunity. And there is the complete removal of disadvantage in practice, which is equality of result. This is not an exhaustive classification but it represents some of the main features of egalitarianism in practice.

The argument for equality of treatment is an argument for treatment without favour, without prejudice. This could mean neutrality between people; but it can also be extended, as Dworkin suggests, to treatment within a particular framework of values.[11] Titmuss, for example, argued:

> There should be no sense of inferiority, pauperism, shame or stigma in the use of a publicly provided service: no attribution that one was being or becoming a 'public burden'. Hence the emphasis on the social rights of all citizens to use or not to use as responsible people the services made available by the community.[12]

Equal treatment does not mean the same treatment: as Benn and Peters comment, 'we should not wish rheumatic patients to be treated like diabetics'.[13]

The second main form of equality is equality of opportunity. The idea was discussed before in the context of liberal individualism. The distinction was made there between prospect- and means-regarding concepts.[14] For equal prospects, there must be competition on equal terms; but competition without disadvantage calls for equal resources. In the former sense, equality of opportunity is simply equivalent to equal treatment; in the latter, it means that people should have what Schaar calls 'the basic conditions necessary for the fullest participation in public life'.[15]

The aim of equality of opportunity is, however, a limited one. The opportunities created are often opportunities to be unequal, and the existence of inequality perpetuates the disadvantages of the lower status groups. If the purpose of equal opportunity is to establish minimum standards for the whole population, it is necessary to consider greater equality not only of opportunity but also of result.

Equal results may be pursued through a number of strategies: Rae outlines four.[16] The first is *maximin*, maximising the minimum. This implies the raising of minimum standards – standards of housing, levels of income, levels of education and health care. This could be done either through selective or universal policies. The second is to address the *ratio* of inequality, increasing the resources of those who are worst off relative to those who are best off. Education and child-related benefits have this effect, even though they distribute more to households on higher incomes. Third, equality may aim for the *least difference*, reducing the range of inequality. Education does not have this effect; age-related benefits do. The fourth is *minimax*, or reducing the advantage of those who are most privileged – private education which gives an advantage to some in competition for places in higher education or the job market, private health care which allows some people to be treated at the cost of delay to others, or the privileges associated with high incomes.

The different approaches to equality – equality of treatment, of opportunity and result – do represent a progressively extending commitment to intervention. Each is motivated by the same guiding principle – the desire to remove disadvantage – though they differ in the extent and scope with which they prevent or compensate for it.

The structure of disadvantage

The structure of disadvantage is often seen in simplistic terms: society continues to be unequal. There are, of course, fluctuations in the structure of inequality – inequality can be more or less dispersed, the top or the bottom can be extended – but for those who (like Marxists) argue that it is the core relationships which matters, these fluctuations may not appear to be of very great importance. There is an extensive literature on inequalities in health and health care, for example, which seems to show that, in the course of forty years, inequalities between social classes have not diminished and may conceivably have widened.[17]

This kind of approach disguises, however, some important shifts in the pattern of relationships. If the problems were the problems of a single class before, they are not now. There is, in industrial societies, a high degree of social mobility – not so high as to lead to immediate and unpredictable reversals of fortune for the mass of people, but certainly high enough to affect the generalisations which can be made. We know, for example, that poor children are more vulnerable to problems and disadvantage than other children, but it is still true that most poor children do not grow up to be poor adults. We know from social research that disadvantage is not passed down from generation to generation, despite the popular myth to the contrary; the effect of the changes in individual circumstances over a lifetime, changing economic fortunes and intermarriage is substantially to erode the numbers of people who are disadvantaged over time.[18]

Most people are not affected continuously by disadvantage. Poverty and disadvantage certainly weight the scales against a person, but they do so for relatively limited periods at any one time. Evidence from Germany suggests that only one poor child in 200 will be poor after five years; the comparable figure for the USA is one child in 500.[19] This does not mean that the numbers of poor people will reduce, because they may well be replaced by other people who will be poor in their turn. Nor should the importance of one person in 500 be under-estimated: where sufficient numbers are affected, this can still refer to tens of thousands of people. It is clear enough, that since poverty is not persistent, there is no basis to suppose a persistent culture or pattern of behaviour associated with poverty.

At the same time, the fluctuating nature of deprivation also means that many people will at some point have some experience of it, for example through a period of unemployment, single parenthood or sickness. The situations in which people are vulnerable have changed. The formerly secure working class involved in manufacturing industries have found themselves highly vulnerable to economic changes; many workers in service industries have found themselves either required to work as independent contractors or as labour for hire, rather than in secure employment. In Europe, the term 'new poor' is being used to describe the situation of people who have been dislocated in the course of economic restructuring. The term calls for a little scepticism, because the new poor experience much the same kind of problems that poor people have always experienced: John Veit Wilson's acerbic comment on the French literature is that 'the only thing that's "new" about this stuff is these people's awareness of it'.[20]

Poverty and exclusion

The idea of poverty is generally used to refer to conditions in which people have limited resources or they experience deprivation, while exclusion refers to the related problems of inequality and social isolation. Neither poverty nor exclusion, however, is a simple term with a clear, agreed meaning. Poverty might be taken to refer to the absence of basic necessities,[21] a lack of resources in itself, or the experience of vulnerability and lack of security which goes with the lack of resources. It may refer specifically to multiple deprivations, a constellation of problems associated with lack of resources and experienced over time. Baratz and Grigsby, for example, point to the characteristic problems of poverty as including a lack of physical comfort, a severe lack of health, a severe lack of safety and security, a lack of 'welfare values' relating to status and social position, and a lack of 'deference values' relating to the structure of power.[22] Research on the pattern of vulnerability to poverty has argued that poverty consists not of a single, unvarying problem or set of problems, but rather of a fluctuating set of conditions characterised by the systematic relationship of the deprivations experienced.[23]

Poverty can also, however, be understood in relational terms – as a special kind of social position in which poor people are disadvantaged relative to others. Poverty has been described in terms of dependency – Simmel identified 'the poor' strongly with the recipients of welfare[24] – and as the experience of inequality:

> There is an inescapable connection between poverty and inequality: certain degrees or dimensions of inequality . . . will lead to people being below the minimum standards acceptable in that society. It is this 'economic distance' aspect of inequality that is poverty.[25]

The idea of 'exclusion' builds on the relational elements, and in the discourse of the European Union it has come to stand for the issues of poverty.

> For some years now we have used the terms 'marginalisation' and 'social exclusion' to denote the severest forms of poverty. Marginalization describes people living on the edge of society whilst the socially excluded have been shut out completely from conventional social norms.[26]

Exclusion, however, is based in a different paradigm from poverty. The idea was popularised in France, where the key concept is the idea of solidarity, referring to a set of social networks in which people would be obligated to each other. People were excluded if they were not part of these networks. Lenoir's influential book, *Les Exclus*, claimed that one person in ten in France was excluded;[27] this led to the development of policies designed to extend the scope of social protection and offer scope for reintegration, or 'insertion', in society.

The idea of exclusion has been important in two ways. First, it has identified the problems of poverty as part of a set of problems of social integration, along with other situations in which people might also be unable to participate fully in society – problems such as racial disadvantage or stigmatisation through illness or disability. Second, it points to a set of strategies. Whereas policies for poverty have tended to be concerned with the provision of material resources, policies for insertion have emphasised the importance of social relationships. The provision of the basic means-tested benefit in France, the *Revenu Minimum d'Insertion*, is conditional on the formation of a contract for insertion, negotiated by recipients with social workers.[28] Many contracts are concerned with employment, because for many people employment is the principal route through which social integration may be achieved, but contracts may also be concerned with family or domestic issues, housing, health and education. For some, the contract is a meaningless form; for others, it represents a very substantial added element to their social protection, covering provision of training courses, skills development or physical facilities. The idea has been influential in the European Union; similar schemes have been introduced in some European countries, and the protocol to the Maastricht Treaty makes specific provision for directives, binding on member states, relating to action against exclusion.

Other forms of inequality

Poverty and exclusion are particularly important from the point of view of social welfare, because both are pervasive conditions which imply a denial of welfare. They are not, however, the only forms of inequality or disadvantage in society, and in some of the previous chapters, particularly Chapter 11, we have considered other forms of disadvantage, which include issues of race, gender and sexuality. Although any of these may make a person vulnerable to poverty or exclusion, they are not sufficient to explain poverty or exclusion in themselves. Women are not generally excluded (their problem is different – they tend to occupy inferior positions within social structures). Most women, and most people in racial minorities are not poor. People in racial minorities and people whose sexuality differs from the norm may in different ways be excluded, but the context of exclusion is often limited and they may well have alternative social networks.

Concern with these issues has shifted the discussion of equality, particularly in the USA and the UK, towards a discussion of the disadvantage of social groups. This depends not on the consideration of the position of individuals but on the relative position of one social group when set against another: Rae describes it as 'bloc-regarding' rather than 'individual-regarding' equality.[29] The terms 'affirmative action' and 'positive discrimination' have come to stand for corrective action intended to reestablish the position of one group against another, which may mean that the interests of the most favoured members of that group are furthered – sometimes in preference to the least favoured. Opposition to the glass ceiling, which prevents women from gaining top positions, is based in the idea that women from higher social classes should be given the same access to privilege as men from the same classes. The desire to ensure that African Americans qualify as doctors or lawyers is not mainly directed at the conditions of poor African Americans, but at the more privileged African Americans. The advocates of these positions sometimes argue, implausibly, that benefits will trickle down to other members of the oppressed category;[30] more convincingly, the argument can simply be made that since existing disadvantages are illegitimate, at least some of them can be removed.

There are powerful objections to these arguments, reviewed for example by John Edwards.[31] Their effect on egalitarian policies has been disturbingly negative, discrediting important arguments on inequality by dogmatic absurdities, distracting attention from the fundamental issues of poverty and exclusion (often with the insistence that the blocs subsume these issues, which they do not). In the case of race in particular, several of the arguments buy into the offensive stereotypes and myths they are supposed to be chal-lenging – that racial minorities have a common experience deter-mined by skin colour, that people's psychology is dominated by their racial characteristics, or that people in racial minorities are poor and dependent. It is important, however, not to lose sight of two moral precepts. One is the argument of liberal individualism, that we must seek to protect the position of each and every person, and that can only happen if each and every person has rights which protect that person from illegitimate disadvantage. The second is the socialist argument that society can and should be judged in moral terms and, that if social processes generate dis-advantage even through processes which are legitimate in them-selves, there is no necessary reason to accept the consequences. On this basis, action to redress the inequalities experienced by people from a range of groups may be both legitimate and desirable.

Social welfare and social justice

Social welfare is intrinsically redistributive, in the sense that those who pay are not the same as those who receive services, and it can be seen as a powerful instrument for the legitimation of redistribution. The redistributive elements can be unpredictable, and some of the literature is devoted to an analysis of the implications of different kinds of measures on the final distribution of welfare: the argument has been made, for example, that subsidies for public transport have a regressive effect,[32] and that facilities for leisure tend to favour the middle classes.[33] Titmuss's famous arguments on the social division of welfare were concerned to draw attention to the complex and sometimes concealed effects of different mechanisms on the distribution of welfare.[34]

Welfare can be seen as having many possible objectives, however, and social justice is only one of them. In the previous chapters, we have considered a range of accounts of the role and function of welfare services including, for example, the promotion of individual welfare, the reproduction of society and the maintenance of social order. The most important objective in Europe is probably social protection, the principle that people should not be exposed by changing fortune to hardship or suffering. This principle, closely allied to the development of social insurance, is central to the development of health services, pensions, unemployment provision and compensation for disability. In most European countries, the protection which is offered is geared to the contributions a person will have made, and so to a person's work record and current level of income. The rights which people have are particular – that is, special to each individual – rather than universal, or available to all.

A second major principle is the aim of social integration, generally understood in terms of solidarity but equally implying some alteration in social relationships. Boulding described integration as an attempt 'to build the identity of a person around some community with which he is associated'.[35] A UN definition of a social service describes it as 'an organized activity that aims at helping towards a mutual adjustment of individuals and their social environment.'[36] Integration in this sense has a double edge: it may be a call for an alteration of a society to meet the needs of the person, but equally (and perhaps more likely) it also implies that people have to be adjusted to fit the society. Although this approach has had little direct influence in the UK or the USA, it has proved to be of great importance in France and, from there, in the European Union.

Third, social welfare services can be seen as promoting welfare, in the general economic sense of material prosperity. The German *Sozialstaat* is devoted to the service of the economic system, which is seen as the mainspring from which welfare can be delivered. Economic development can be promoted directly, through the provision of services which facilitate the operations of the economic process – employment and labour market policies, or housing for workers; and, indirectly, by developing conditions which favour economic development – the protection of the health of the workforce, or their education. Much of the Marxist analysis depends on extending the principle of co-operation with industry to the point where it becomes the dominant part of its *raison d'être*.

Although this is far from a full consideration of the aims of welfare provision[37] it is enough to point to a central conceptual problem in the pursuit of social justice: that, whatever justice may be, and however it is understood, it cannot be sufficient in itself to determine the aims or justify the outcomes of social policies. This is why advocates of social equality, like Tawney or Crosland, do not even try to argue for an equal society, or for a just one. They argue only for more justice, and more equality, than we have at present. True equality may be, Tawney commented, impossible, but the impossibility of absolute cleanliness is no reason to roll around in a dungheap.[38]

The future of welfare

From the perspective of the UK, the existence of welfare services seems at times to be under threat. The welfare state which was founded in the post-war period was supposedly built on principles of universality, with a strong focus on provision by the state. The model which traditionally opposed this was the model of the old Poor Law: the provision of welfare as a public burden, on a residual basis, offered at the lowest level possible, with the normal expectation being that people would provide through the private sector to meet their needs, rather than relying on the state. The constellation of views which this represents has led to a strong association of residualism with inadequate benefits and penal attitudes to the poor. The effect of moving to private services, and the residualisation of key services such as public housing and income maintenance, is seen by many as a sign of the end of the welfare state. Certainly, the acceptance of the principle that old people would be required to contribute to long-stay residential care was represented in the British press as 'the end of the welfare state', an abandonment of the promise that welfare would be provided 'from cradle to grave'.[39]

The European experience suggests a different interpretation. Most of the European welfare states have never had the explicit commitment to universality which characterised the British model, but rather have based welfare on the progressive extension of particular rights. They have not been geared solely, or even primarily, to the provision of services by the state, but have developed a range of provisions provided by autonomous, or quasi-autonomous, funds – an arrangement which has often, as it has turned out, proved more robust politically than provision by the state. They have been concerned less with redistribution than with social protection and yet, despite this, have often proved to be at least as effective in their redistributive outcomes as the British system. Although the British welfare state has been very effective in certain respects – particularly in relation to health care, where it has provided economical care on a universal basis – in other respects, and most clearly in relation to provision for pensions and unemployment, the British approach has been weighed in the balance and found wanting. Privatisation and the development of particular benefits in relation to pensions do not mark a return to the principles of the Poor Law but, rather, reflect the failure of the Beveridge scheme relative to Bismarckian, or at least to other European, systems of social insurance.

Within the European welfare states, it seems that the principle of social protection has come to dominate over the ideal of social justice. Social justice calls for an ordered, patterned structure in the distribution of goods and resources. Social protection calls for intervention in a way which leaves the initial distribution of resources unchanged – a principle which often means that more resources go to richer people, because rich people have further to fall. The popularity of social protection is that it offers security in an insecure environment, and security is important for everyone – for middle-class people because they have a lot to lose, and for poor people because they are likely to lose the little they have.[40]

The apparent erosion of the institutional ideal may, then, be a side issue. The main test of the durability of welfare is not whether it continues to be provided by the state, and not even whether it makes society more equal, but whether the collective provision of welfare continues to be a mechanism through which issues of welfare, legitimacy, distribution, social integration and social protection are addressed. This is the position which was so vigorously opposed by the radical right, who argued that government had no business addressing any of these issues; equally, the position was discounted by Marxists, who accepted that welfare might be used in some of these ways, but held that it was incapable of redressing the balance. The provision of welfare has been so far institutionalised in developed economies as to be inseparable from their operation, and only the most radical change in those societies would have the potential to challenge its role.

Notes

I Introduction: thinking about society

1 K. Popper, 1968, *The Logic of Scientific Discovery*, London: Hutchinson.
2 M. Oakeshott, 1975, The vocabulary of a modern European state, *Political Studies*, 23(2–3), 319–41.
3 I.M.D. Little, 1957, *A Critique of Welfare Economics*, 2nd edn, Oxford: Oxford University Press.
4 E. Goffman, 1959, *The Presentation of Self in Everyday Life*, Harmondsworth: Penguin Books, 1971.
5 R. Dahrendorf, 1973, *Homo Sociologicus*, London: Routledge and Kegan Paul.
6 D. Wrong, 1967, The oversocialised conception of man in modern sociology, in H.J. Demerath and R. Peterson (eds), *System Change and Conflict*, New York: Free Press.
7 P. Berger and T. Luckmann, 1967, *The Social Construction of Reality*, New York: Anchor.
8 E. Burke, 1790, *Reflections on the Revolution in France*, New York: Holt, Rinehart and Winston, 1959.
9 H. Wilensky and C. Lebeaux, 1958, *Industrial Society and Social Welfare*, New York: Free Press, 1965.
10 G. Esping-Andersen, 1990, *The Three Worlds of Welfare Capitalism*, Cambridge: Polity.
11 F. Castles, 1994, Comparing the Australian and Scandinavian welfare States, *Scandinavian Political Studies*, 17(1), 31–46.
12 B. Cass and J. Freeland, 1994, Social security and full employment in Australia, in J. Hills, J. Ditch and H. Glennerster (eds) *Beveridge and Social Security*, Oxford: Clarendon Press.
13 For example, R. Albon and D. Stafford, 1987, *Rent Control*, Beckenham: Croom Helm.
14 L. Althusser, 1969, *For Marx*, Harmondsworth: Penguin.
15 J.J. Rousseau, 1762, The social contract, in E. Barker (ed.), 1971, *Social Contract*, Oxford: Oxford University Press, opening sentence.
16 U. Beck, 1992, *Risk Society*, London: Sage.

2 Keynesian economics

1 Keynes' letter to Bernard Shaw of 6 January 1935.
2 J. Robinson, 1986, *The Economics of Keynes*, Harmondsworth: Penguin, p. 320.
3 Robinson, 1986, p.258.
4 A. Smith, 1776, *The Wealth of Nations*, London: Everyman's.
5 A.C. Pigou, 1933, *The Theory of Unemployment*, London: Macmillan.
6 J.M. Keynes, 1936, *The General Theory of Employment, Interest and Money*, London: Macmillan, p.129.
7 G. Davidson and P. Davidson, 1988, *Economics in a Civilised Society*, London: Macmillan, p.20.
8 Keynes, 1936, p.129.
9 Keynes, 1936, p.129.
10 A. Phillips, 1958, The relationship between unemployment and the rate of change of money wage rates in the UK 1861–1957, *Economica*, 25, 283–99.
11 P. Ormerod, 1994, On inflation and unemployment, in J. Michie and J. Grieve Smith (eds), *Unemployment in Europe*, London: Academic Press, p.53.
12 M. Friedman, 1975, *Unemployment versus Inflation: An Evaluation of the Phillips Curve*, Sussex: Institute of Economic Affairs.
13 J.M. Keynes, 1944, A note by Lord Keynes, *Economic Journal*, December, 429.
14 Keynes in Lord Kahn, 1974, On re-reading Keynes, *Proceedings of the British Academy*, IX, 371.
15 A. Echner, 1979, *A Guide to Post-Keynesian Economics*, London: Macmillan, p.175.
16 Ormerod, 1994.
17 G. Therborn, 1986, *Why Some People are More Unemployed Than Others*, London: Verso.
18 Therborn, 1986, p.132.
19 Cited in T. Watkins, 1995, *The Oxfam Poverty Report*, Oxford: Oxfam, p.72.
20 Watkins, 1995, pp.75–6.
21 Keynes, 1936, p.383.
22 Keynes, 1936, p.372.
23 D. Bell, 1965, *The End of Ideology*, 2nd edn, New York: Free Press.
24 P.C. Schmitter, 1979, Still the century of corporatism?, in P.C. Schmitter and G. Lehmbruch (eds), *Trends towards Corporatist Intermediation*, Beverly Hills: Sage, p.13.
25 P. Bachrach and M.S. Baratz, 1970, *Power and Poverty: Theory and Practice*, Oxford: Oxford University Press.

3 Marxism

1 K. Marx and F. Engels, 1848/1967, *The Communist Manifesto*, Harmondsworth: Penguin.

2　K. Marx, Preface to A contribution to the critique of political economy, in *Karl Marx and Frederick Engels: Selected Works*, London: Lawrence and Wishart, 1968, p.181.

3　Marx, Engels, 1848/1967.

4　K. Popper, 1945, *The Open Society and its Enemies, Vol. 2*, London: George Routledge, pp.127–8.

5　C.A.R. Crosland, 1956, *The Future of Socialism*, London: Cape.

6　W. Kymlicka, 1990, *Contemporary Political Philosophy*, Oxford: Clarendon, pp.176–7.

7　K. Marx, 1875, Critique of the Gotha Programme, in *Karl Marx and Frederick Engels, Selected Works*, London: Lawrence and Wishart, 1968.

8　P. Saunders, 1979, *Urban Politics*, Harmondsworth: Penguin, p.147.

9　C. Offe, *Contradictions of the Welfare State*, London: Hutchinson.

10　Offe, 1984, p.263.

11　K. Marx, 1912, The general law of capitalist accumulation, *Capital, Vol. 2*, London: William Glaisher, Ch. 25.

12　Marx, 1912.

13　S. Samad, 1994, Asian chapter in *The Study of Poverty in North America*, CROP/UNESCO symposium on regional state-of-the-art reviews on poverty research, Paris.

14　F. Engels, 1934, *Anti-Dühring*, London: Lawrence and Wishart, p.121.

15　R.H. Tawney, 1931, *Equality*, London: Allen and Unwin.

16　See e.g. E. Wilson, 1977, *Women and the Welfare State*, London: Tavistock.

17　H. Hartmann, 1995, The unhappy marriage of marxism and feminism, in D. Tallack (ed.) *Critical theory: A Reader*, New York: Harvester Wheatsheaf.

18　e.g. E. Laclau and C. Mouffe, 1985, *Hegemony and Socialist Strategy*, London: Verso.

19　Marx, Engels, 1848, p.82.

20　R. Miliband, 1969, *The State in Capitalist Society*, London: Weidenfeld and Nicolson.

21　N. Poulantzas, 1978, *State, Power, Socialism*, trans. P. Camiller, NLB, London: pp.184–5.

22　J. O'Connor, 1973, *The Fiscal Crisis of the State*, New York: St. Martin's Press, pp.150–1.

23　J. Habermas, 1976, *Legitimation Crisis*, London: Heinemann, p.35.

24　Offe, 1984, p.153.

25　A.B. Atkinson, 1995, *The Welfare State and Economic Performance*, London: London School of Economics/Suntory-Toyota Centre for Economics and Related Disciplines.

26　S. Spitzer, 1975, Toward a Marxian theory of deviance, *Social Problems*, 22(5), 638–51.

27　P. Spicker, 1988, *Principles of Social Welfare*, London: Routledge.

28　See Organisation for Economic Co-operation and Development, 1990, *Health Care Systems in Transition*, Paris: OECD; and OECD, 1992, *The Reform of Health Care*, Paris: OECD.

4 Liberal individualism

1 R. Nozick, 1974, *Anarchy, State and Utopia*, Oxford: Blackwell, p.ix.
2 H. Thorea, 1854, Walden, in C. Bode (ed.), *The Portable Thoreau*, New York: Viking Press, 1947.
3 R. Nozick, 1984, Moral constraints and distributive justice, in M. Sandel (ed.), *Liberalism and its Critics*, Oxford: Blackwell, p.105.
4 J. Locke, 1690, *Two Treatises of Civil Government*, (P. Laslett, ed.), 1965, New York: Mentor, p.346.
5 D. Rae, 1981, *Equalities*, Cambridge, Mass.: Harvard University Press, p.47.
6 F. Hayek, 1984, Value and merit, in M. Sandel (ed.), p.80.
7 J. Pahl, 1989, *Money and Marriage*, London: Macmillan.
8 S. Shaver, 1993/1994, Body rights, social rights and the liberal welfare state, *Critical Social Policy*, 39, 66–93.
9 D. Rae, 1981, *Equalities*, Cambridge, Mass.: Harvard University Press.
10 F. Hayek and W. Bartley, 1988, *The Fatal Conceit*, London: Routledge, p.9.
11 Nozick, 1974.
12 C. Kukathas, 1990, *Hayek and Modern Liberalism*, Oxford: Clarendon Press.
13 F. Hayek, 1976, *Law, Legislation and Liberty, Vol. 2: The Mirage of Social Justice*, London: Routledge and Kegan Paul.
14 C. Taylor, 1979, What's wrong with negative liberty? in A. Ryan (ed.), *The Idea of Freedom*, Oxford: Oxford University Press.
15 Nozick, 1974.
16 D. Green, 1987, *The New Right*, Brighton: Harvester Wheatsheaf.
17 A. Smith, 1776, *The Wealth of Nations*, London: Everyman's 1991 edn, p.13.
18 S. Brittan, 1982, in *The Financial Times*, 16 September.
19 J. Schumpeter, 1967, Two concepts of democracy, in A. Quinton (ed.), *Political Philosophy*, Oxford: Oxford University Press.
20 A. Downs, 1957, *An Economic Theory of Democracy*, New York: Harper and Row.
21 S. Brittan, 1977, *The Economic Consequences of Democracy*, London: Temple Smith.
22 Green, 1987.
23 S. Beer, 1982, *Britain against Itself*, London: Faber and Faber.
24 J. Le Grand, 1997, Knights, knaves or pawns? *Journal of Social Policy*, 26(2), 149–70.
25 J. Le Grand and W. Bartlett, 1993, *Quasi-markets and Social Policy*, Basingstoke: Macmillan.

5 Conservatism and the New Right

1 A. Gewirth (ed.), 1979, *Marsilius of Padua*, New York: Arno.
2 F.H. Bradley, 1876, *Ethical Studies*, London.
3 S. Beer, 1982, *Modern British Politics*, London: Faber.
4 N. Coote, 1989, Catholic social teaching, *Social Policy and Administration*, 23(2).

5 Lord Halifax, 1684, The character of a timmer, in J.P. Kenyon (ed.), 1969, *Halifax: Complete Works*, Harmondsworth: Penguin.
6 E. Burke, 1790, *Reflections on the Revolution in France*, New York: Holt, Rinehart and Winston, 1959 edn, p.72.
7 Burke, 1790, p.23.
8 K. Mannheim, 1936, *Ideology and Utopia*, trans. I. Wirth and E. Shils, London: Routledge and Kegan Paul.
9 Pius XI, 1931, *Quadragesimo Anno, Actae Apostolicae Sedis*, 23, p.203.
10 Pius XI, 1931, p.203.
11 Commission of the European Communities, 1993, *Commission Report to the European Council on the Adaptation of Community Legislation to the Subsidiarity Principle*, COM(93) 545 final Brussels, 24.11.93.
12 Pius XI, 1931, p.203.
13 J. Delors, 1991, *Le principe de subsidiarité: contribution au débat*, Maastricht: Colloque de l'Institut Européen d'administration publique, s.I.
14 Reported in *Il Resto del Carlino*, March 1992, Bologna.
15 A. Kuyper, 1899, *Calvinism: Six Stone Lectures*, Amsterdam: Höveker and Wormser, p.116.
16 Kuyper, 1899, p.118.
17 See P. Marshall, 1985, Dooyeweerd's empirical theory of rights, in C.T. McIntyre (ed.), *The Legacy of Herman Dooyeweerd*, Lanham: University Press of America.
18 M. Pijl, 1993, The Dutch Welfare State, in R. Page and J. Baldock (eds), *Social Policy Review 5*, SPA.

6 Social democracy and socialism

1 *The Federalist Papers*, 1787–88, New York: New American Library, 1961.
2 R. Owen, 1927, *A New View of Society*, London: Dent.
3 T.H. Marshall, 1981, *The Right to Welfare*, London: Heinemann.
4 T.H. Marshall, 1963, *Sociology at the Crossroads*, London: Heinemann, p.87.
5 M. Bulmer and A. Rees, 1996, *Citizenship Today*, London: UCL Press.
6 H. Wilensky and C. Lebeaux, 1958/1965, *Industrial Society and Social Welfare*, New York: Free Press.
7 R.M. Titmuss, 1974, *Social Policy: An Introduction*, London: George Allen and Unwin.
8 R. Mishra, 1981, *Society and Social Policy*, 2nd edn, London: Macmillan.
9 G. MacCallum, 1967, Negative and positive freedom, *Philosophical Review*, 76, 312–34.
10 R.H. Tawney, 1931, *Equality*, London: Unwin, 1964, p.107.
11 Tawney, 1931, p.52.
12 D. Rae, 1981, *Equalities*, Cambridge, Mass.: Harvard University Press.
13 R. Nozick, 1974, *Anarchy, State and Utopia*, Oxford: Blackwell.
14 P. Spicker, 1991, Solidarity, in G. Room (ed.), *Towards a European Welfare State?*, Bristol: SAUS, pp.17–37.
15 R.M. Titmuss, 1970, *The Gift Relationship*, Harmondsworth: Penguin.

16 Tawney, 1931, p.122.
17 J. Le Grand, 1982, *The Strategy of Equality*, London: George Allen and Unwin.

7 Communities and society

1 A. MacIntyre, 1981, *After Virtue: A Study in Moral Theory*, London: Duckworth, pp.204–5.
2 D. Clarke, 1975, The Conservative faith in a modern age, in P.W. Buck (ed.), *How Conservatives Think*, Harmondsworth: Penguin, p.166.
3 J. Charvet, 1983, The idea of equality as a substantive principle of society, in W. Letwin (ed.), *Against Equality*, London: Macmillan.
4 M. Walzer, 1984, Welfare, membership and need, in M. Sandel (ed.), *Liberalism and its Critics*, Oxford: Blackwell, p.205.
5 M. Maimonides, 1180, The eight degrees of benevolence, in M. Maimonides and I. Ibn Al-Nakawa, *The Degrees of Jewish Benevolence*, Society of Jewish Bibliophiles, 1964.
6 M. Luther, 1536, Ordinance for a common chest, in F.R. Salter (ed.), 1926, *Some Early Tracts on Poor Relief*, London: Methuen.
7 Cited N. Coote, 1989, Catholic Social Teaching, *Social Policy and Administration* 23(2), 157.
8 E. Alfarandi, 1989, *Action et aide sociales*, Paris: Dalloz, 4th edn, p.73.
9 A.W. Gouldner, 1960, The norm of reciprocity, *American Sociological Review*, 25(2), 161–77.
10 G.C. Homans, 1961, *Social Behaviour*, London: Routledge and Kegan Paul.
11 P.M. Blau, 1964, *Exchange and Power in Social Life*, New York: John Wiley and Sons.
12 R. Pinker, 1971, *Social Theory and Social Policy*, London: Heinemann, Ch. 4.
13 M. Mauss, 1925, *The Gift*, London: Cohen and West, 1966.
14 R.M. Titmuss, 1970, *The Gift Relationship*, Harmondsworth: Penguin.
15 M. Sahlins, 1974, *Stone-age Economics*, London: Tavistock.
16 E. Durkheim, 1915, *The Division of Labour in Society*, New York: Free Press, 1964.
17 R.M. Titmuss, 1955, The social division of welfare: some reflections on the search for equity, in *Essays on 'the Welfare State'*, 2nd edn 1963, London: George Allen and Unwin; see P. Spicker, 1984, Titmuss's social division of welfare: a reappraisal, in C. Jones and J. Stevenson (eds), *Yearbook of Social Policy in Britain 1983*, London: RKP.
18 C. Offe, 1984, *Contradictions of the Welfare State*, London: Hutchinson.
19 T. Parsons, 1952, *The Social System*, London: Tavistock; R. Merton, 1968, *Social Theory and Social Structure*, New York: Free Press, 3rd edn.
20 C. Lévi-Strauss, 1949, *The Elementary Structures of Kinship*, trans. J.H. Bell, J.R. von Sturmer and R. Needham, rev. edn 1969, London: Eyre and Spottiswoode.
21 T. Parsons, 1966, *Societies: Evolutionary and Comparative Perspectives*, Englewood Cliffs: Prentice Hall.

22 M. Haralambos and M. Holborn, 1991, *Sociology: Themes and Perspectives*, London: Collins, p.780.
23 D. Lee and H. Newby, 1983, *The Problem of Sociology*, London: Hutchinson, p.271.
24 T. Parsons, 1969, *Politics and Social Structure*, New York: Free Press.
25 e.g. T. Parsons, 1958, Definitions of health and illness, in E.G. Jaco (ed.), *Patients, Physicians and Illness*, Glenco: Free Press.
26 T. Parsons, 1965, Full citizenship for the Negro American?, *Daedalus*, 94, November.
27 See Commissariat général du plan, 1993, *Cohésion sociale et prévention de l'exclusion*, Paris: La Documentation Française.
28 S. Tiemann, 1993, Opinion on social exclusion, *Official Journal of the European Communities*, 93/C 352/13, p.37.
29 Commission of the European Communities, 1992, *Towards a Europe of Solidarity*, COM (92) 542 final, p.8.

8 New views of the economy

1 J.K. Galbraith, 1972, *The New Industrial State*, rev. edn, Harmondsworth: Penguin.
2 B. Jessop, 1994, Post-fordism and the state, in A. Amin (ed.), *Post-Fordism: A Reader*, Oxford: Blackwell.
3 S. Hall, cited A. Amin, 1994, Post-fordism, in A. Amin (ed.), *Post-Fordism: A Reader*, Oxford, Blackwell, p.31.
4 See R. Burrows and B. Loader (eds), 1994, *Towards a Post-Fordist Welfare State?*, London: Routledge.
5 C. Sabel, 1989, Flexible specialisation and the re-emergence of regional economies, in P. Hirst and J. Zeitlin (eds), *Reversing Industrial Decline?*, Oxford: Berg.
6 D. Matza and H. Miller, 1976, Poverty and proletariat, in R.K. Merton and R. Nisbet (eds), *Contemporary Social Problems*, New York: Harcourt Brace Jovanovich, 4th edn, pp.661–2.
7 For example, A. Seldon, 1977, *Charge!*, London: Temple Smith; P. Minford, M. Peel and P. Ashton, 1987, *The Housing Morass*, London: Institute of Economic Affairs.
8 J. Rex and R. Moore, 1967, *Race, Community and Conflict*, Oxford: Oxford University Press.
9 P. Saunders, 1986, *Social Theory and the Urban Question*, London: Hutchinson.
10 M. Cahill, 1994, *The New Social Policy*, Oxford: Blackwell.
11 M. Ferrera, 1996, The 'Southern Model' of welfare in social Europe, *Journal of European Social Policy*, 6(1), 17–37.

9 The global economy

1 Cited in D. Pepper, 1993, *Eco-socialism*, London: Routledge, p.142.
2 U.N.: United Nations General Assembly, 1991, *International Cooperation for the Eradication of Poverty in Developing Countries*. Report by the Secretary General. Document A/46/454.

3 R. Mishra, 1994, *The Study of Poverty in North America*, CROP/ UNESCO symposium on regional state-of-the-art reviews on poverty research, Paris.

4 P. Streeten, 1995, Comments on 'The framework of ILO action against poverty', in G. Rodgers (ed.), *The Poverty Agenda and the ILO*, Geneva: International Labour Office.

5 M. Ferrera, 1996, The 'Southern Model' of welfare in social Europe, *Journal of European Social Policy*, 6(1), 17–37.

6 J. Drèze and A. Sen, 1989, *Hunger and Public Action*, Oxford: Clarendon Press.

7 L. Doyal and I. Gough, 1991, *A Theory of Human Need*, London: Macmillan.

8 International Monetary Fund (IMF), 1997, *World Economic Outlook*, p.72.

9 K. Marx and F. Engels, 1848, *The Communist Manifesto*, Harmondsworth: Penguin.

10 D. Harvey, 1989, *The Condition of Postmodernity*, Oxford: Blackwell.

11 P. Hirst and G. Thompson, 1996, *Globalisation in Question*, Brighton: Polity.

12 IMF, 1997, p.13.

13 IMF, 1997, p.5.

14 IMF, 1997, p.13.

15 A. Revenga, 1992, Exporting jobs?: the impact of competition on employment and wages in US manufacturing, *Quarterly Journal of Economics*, 107, 255–84; D. Neven and C. Wyplosz, 1996, *Relative Prices and Restructuring in European Industry*, London: Centre for Policy Research Working Paper no. 1451.

16 IMF, 1997, p.91.

17 K. Deutsch, 1981, From the national welfare state to the international welfare system, in W. Mommsen (ed.), *The Emergence of the Welfare States in Britain and Germany*, Beckenham: Croom Helm.

18 A. de Swaan, 1992, Perspectives for transnational social policy, *Government and Opposition*, 21(1), 33–51.

19 B. Jessop, 1994, Post-fordism and the state, in A. Amin (ed.), *Post Fordism: A Reader*, Oxford: Blackwell.

20 A. de Swaan (ed.), 1994, *Social Policy beyond Borders*, Amsterdam: Amsterdam University Press.

21 P.J. Slot, 1996, Harmonisation, *European Law Review*, 21(5), 378–97.

22 Commission of the European Communities, 1993, Green Paper: *European Social Policy – Options for the Union*, Com (93) final; Commission of the European Communities 1994, White Paper: *European Social Policy – a Way Forward for the Union*, Com (93) 333 final.

23 P. Spicker, 1991, The principle of subsidiarity and the social policy of the European Community, *Journal of European Social Policy*, 1(1), 3–14.

24 P. Spicker, 1997, The prospect for European laws on poverty, in A. Kjonstad and J. Veit-Wilson (eds), *Law, Power and Poverty*, Bergen: Comparative Research Programme on Poverty.

25 Y. Chassard and O. Quintin, 1992, Social protection in the European Community: towards a convergence of policies, a paper presented to the International Conference on Social Security 50 years after Beveridge, University of York.
26 M. Ferrera, 1996, The 'Southern Model' of welfare in social Europe, *Journal of European Social Policy*, 6(1), 17–37.

10 A new kind of society

1 N.J. Rengger, 1995, *Political Theory, Modernity and Postmodernity*, Oxford: Blackwell.
2 S. White, 1994, *Political Theory and Postmodernism*, Cambridge: Cambridge University Press.
3 M. Foucault, 1995, Truth and power, in D. Tallack (ed.), *Critical Theory: A Reader*, New York: Harvester Wheatsheaf, p.69.
4 A. Giddens, 1994, *Beyond Left and Right*, Cambridge: Polity Press.
5 Ibid.
6 A. Giddens, in U. Beck, A. Giddens and S. Lash, 1994, *Reflexive Modernization*, Oxford: Polity Press, p.187.
7 Ibid., pp.174, 182.
8 e.g. J. Moore, 1989, *The End of the Line for Poverty*, London: Conservative Political Centre; N. Dennis, 1996, *The Invention of Permanent Poverty*, London: Institute of Economic Affairs.
9 F. Coffield and J. Sarsby, 1980, *A Cycle of Deprivation?*, London: Heinemann.
10 Z. Bauman, 1995, *Life in Fragments*, Oxford: Blackwell, p.37.
11 U. Beck, 1992, *Risk Society*, London: Sage.
12 J. Burnet, 1989, *Plenty and Want*, London: Routledge.
13 U. Beck, 1997, *Reinventing Politics*, Oxford: Polity Press, p.95.
14 Beck, 1997, p.97.
15 Z. Bauman, 1997, *Postmodernity and its Discontents*, Oxford: Blackwell, p.200.
16 Bauman, 1997, p.202.
17 A. Giddens, 1991, *Modernity and Self Identity*, Cambridge: Polity Press, p.231.
18 W. Connolly, 1991, *Identity/Difference*, London: Cornell University Press.
19 P. Hansen, 1993, *Hannah Arendt: Politics, History and Citizenship*, Cambridge: Polity Press.
20 M. Foucault in P. Rabinow (ed.), 1984, *The Foucault Reader*, Harmondsworth: Penguin, pp.383–4.
21 P. Taylor Gooby, 1994, Postmodernism and social policy: a great leap backwards, *Journal of Social Policy*, 23(3), 385–404.

11 Explaining social divisions

1 B. Disraeli, 1845, *Sybil or The Two Nations*, Harmondsworth: Penguin, 1980.

2 T.W. Adorno, E. Frenkel-Brunswick, D.J. Levinson and R.N. Sanford, 1950, *The Authoritarian Personality*, New York: W.W. Norton and Co., 1969.

3 E. Fromm, 1942, *The Fear of Freedom*, London: Kegan Paul.

4 J. Habermas, 1990, Discourse ethics: notes on a program of philosophical justification, in S. Benhabib and F. Dallmayr (eds), *The Communicative Ethics Controversy*, Cambridge: Mass.: MIT Press, pp.68–70.

5 J. Higgins, Social control theories of social policy, *Journal of Social Policy*, 1980, 9(1), 1–23.

6 R. Beerman, 1960, The law against parasites, tramps and beggars, *Soviet Studies*, 11(4), 453–5.

7 S. Lukes, 1978, Power and authority, in T. Bottomore and R. Nisbet (eds), *A History of Sociological Analysis*, London: Heinemann.

8 P. Bourdieu and J. Passeron, 1977, *Reproduction in Education, Society and Culture*, London: Sage.

9 S. Sharpe, 1994, *Just Like a Girl*, Harmondsworth: Penguin.

10 M. Foucault, 1976, *Histoire de la sexualité: la volonté de savoir*, Paris: Gallimard, pp.121–2.

11 Foucault, 1976, p.122.

12 Foucault, 1976, pp.123–7.

13 M. Foucault, 1981, The order of discourse in R. Young (ed.), *Untying the Text*, London: Methuen, p.52.

14 S. White, 1994, *Political Theory and Postmodernism*, Cambridge: Cambridge University Press, p.8.

15 M. Foucault, 1975, *Surveiller et punir*, Paris: Gallimard.

16 M. Foucault, 1961, *Madness and Civilisation*, London: Tavistock, 1965.

17 K. Jones, 1993, *Asylums and After*, London: Athlone Press.

18 N. Thompson, 1993, *Anti-discriminatory Practice*, London: Macmillan.

19 P. Freire, 1972, *Pedagogy of the Oppressed*, Harmondsworth: Penguin, p.68.

20 G. Mitchell, 1989, Empowerment and opportunity, *Social Work Today*, 16 March.

21 J. Dalrymple and B. Burke, 1995, *Anti-oppressive Practice*, Buckingham: Open University Press; M. Langan and L. Day (eds), 1993, *Women, Oppression and Social Work*, London: Routledge; A. Mullender and D. Ward, Empowerment and oppression, in J. Walmsley, J. Reynolds, P. Shakespeare and R. Woolfe (eds), 1993, *Health, Welfare and Practice*, London: Sage.

22 Dalrymple and Burke, 1995, p.3.

23 K. Millett, 1977, *Sexual Politics*, London: Virago, esp. Ch. 2.

24 J. Mitchell, 1971, *Women's Estate*, Harmondsworth: Penguin, p.65.

25 C. Delphy, 1984, Sex classes, in S. Jackson *et al.* (eds), 1993, *Women's Studies: A Reader*, New York: Harvester Wheatsheaf.

26 M. Barrett, 1988, *Women's Oppression Today*, London: Verso, pp.249–50.

27 L. Doyal, 1995, *What Makes Women Sick*, Basingstoke: Macmillan, p.4.

28 S. Payne, 1991, *Women, Health and Poverty*, London: Harvester Wheat-sheaf, p.1.
29 G. Pascall, 1986, *Social Policy: A Feminist Analysis*, London: Tavistock, p.27.
30 Pascall, 1986, p.66.
31 Pascall, 1986, p.219.

12 Society

1 E. Evans-Pritchard, 1940, *The Nuer*, Oxford: Oxford University Press.
2 E. Ladurie, 1980, *Montaillou*, Harmondsworth: Penguin.
3 P. Kropotkin, 1939, *Mutual Aid*, Harmondsworth: Penguin.
4 D. Wrong, 1967, The oversocialised conception of man in modern sociology, in H.J. Demerath and R. Peterson (eds), *System Change and Conflict*, New York: Free Press.
5 E. Miller and G. Gwynne, 1972, *A Life Apart*, London: Tavistock, p.80.
6 P. Halmos, 1973, *The Faith of the Counsellors*, London: Constable.
7 B. Compton and B. Galaway, 1973, *Social Work Processes*, Home-wood, Ill.: Dorsey.
8 N. Dennis and C. Erdos, 1992, *Families without Fatherhood*, London: IEA.
9 C. Murray, 1989, *The Emerging British Underclass*, London: Institute of Economic Affairs.
10 N. Dennis, 1996, *The Invention of Permanent Poverty*, London: IEA Health and Welfare Unit.
11 Dennis and Erdos, 1992.
12 R. Lampard, 1994, An examination of the relationship between marital dissolution and unemployment, in D. Gallie, C. Marsh and C. Vogler (eds), *Social Change and the Experience of Unemployment*, Oxford: Oxford University Press.
13 K. Kiernan and V. Estaugh, 1993, research cited in the *Guardian*, Parents who cohabit poorer than those who marry, 1 June, p.4.
14 D. Debordeaux, 1994, Une lecture critique du rapport du CERC: Précarité et risque d'exclusion en France, *Recherches et Prévisions*, 38, 125–34.
15 Kiernan and Estaugh, 1993.
16 C. Murray, 1994, *Underclass: The Crisis Deepens*, Institute of Economic Affairs.
17 C. Murray, 1989, p.27.
18 H. Rodman, 1971, *Lower-class Families: The Culture of Poverty in Negro Trinidad*, London: Oxford University Press.
19 H. Rodman, 1963, The lower-class value stretch, *Social Forces*, 42(2), 205–15.
20 W.J. Wilson, 1987, *The Truly Disadvantaged*, Chicago: University of Chicago Press, pp.90–2; and see Ch. 3.
21 C. Jenks, 1992, *Rethinking Social Policy*, Cambridge: Mass.: Harvard University Press, p.158.
22 R. Jarrett, 1994, Living poor: family life among single parent African American women, *Social Problems*, 41(1), 38.

23 M. Sullivan, 1989, Absent fathers in the inner city, *Annals of the American Academy of Political and Social Science*, 501, 48–58; E. Anderson, 1989, Sex codes and family life among poor inner-city youths, *Annals of the American Academy of Political and Social Science*, 501, 59–78.

24 G. Hillery, 1955, Definitions of community: areas of agreement, *Rural Sociology*, 20, 111–23.

25 e.g. M. Bulmer, 1986, *Social Science and Social Policy*, London: Allen and Unwin.

26 Wilson, 1987.

27 D. Massey, A. Gross and K. Shibuya, 1994, Migration, segregation and the geographic concentration of poverty, *American Sociological Review*, 59(3), 425–45.

28 P. Spicker, 1992, Victorian values, in C. Grant (ed.), *Built to Last?*, London: Roof.

29 A. Coleman, 1985, *Utopia on Trial: Vision and Reality in Planned Housing*, London: Shipman.

30 J. Crane, 1991, Effects of neighbourhoods on dropping out of school and teenage childbearing, in C. Jencks and P. Peterson (eds), *The Urban Underclass*, Washington D.C.: Brookings.

31 R. Lister, 1990, *The Exclusive Society*, London: Child Poverty Action Group; C. Oppenheim, 1990, *Poverty: the Facts*, CPAG, p.15.

32 R. McGahey, cited in Wilson, 1987, p.6.

33 H. Gans, 1990, Deconstructing the underclass, *American Planning Association Journal*, 271, cited in F. Gaffikin and M. Morrissey, 1992, *The New Unemployed*, London: Zed Books, p.84.

34 See e.g. D. Marsden, 1973, *Mothers Alone*, Harmondsworth: Penguin, pp. 136–8, 175–6; or Titmuss and Townsend, cited J. MacNicol, 1987, In pursuit of the underclass, *Journal of Social Policy*, 16(3), 300.

35 e.g. E. Banfield, 1968, *The Unheavenly City*, Boston: Little Brown. See the critique of such work in W. Ryan, 1971, *Blaming the Victim*, London: Orbach and Chambers.

36 K. Auletta, 1983, *The Underclass*, New York: Vintage Books, p.21; C. Murray, 1989, Underclass, *Sunday Times Magazine*, 26 November, 26.

37 A. Neil, 1995, The poor may be richer but the underclass is growing, *Sunday Times*, 28 May, 3–5.

38 D. Matza, 1967, The disreputable poor, in R. Bendix and S.M. Lipset, *Class, Status and Power*, 2nd edn, London: Routledge and Kegan Paul.

39 This is the sense in which the term is used in F. Field, 1989, *Losing Out*, Oxford: Blackwell.

40 M. Bulmer, 1989, The underclass, empowerment and public policy, in M. Bulmer, J. Lewis and D. Piachaud (eds), *The Goals of Social Policy*, London: Unwin Hyman, p.246.

41 J. Rodger, 1992, The welfare state and social closure, *Critical Social Policy*, 35, 45–63, 58.

42 See P. Spicker, 1988, *Principles of Social Welfare*, London: Routledge, Ch. 3.

43 D. Matza and H. Miller, 1976, Poverty and proletariat, in R.K. Merton and R. Nisbet (eds), *Contemporary Social Problems*, New York: Harcourt Brace Jovanovich, 4th edn, pp.661–2.
44 L. Morris and S. Irwin, 1992, Employment histories and the concept of the underclass, *Sociology*, 26(3), 401–20.
45 H.W. Williams, 1944, Benjamin Franklin and the Poor Laws, *Social Service Review*, 18(1), 77–91.
46 Reviewed in Wilson, 1987.
47 C. Murray, 1984, *Losing Ground*, New York: Basic Books.
48 E. McLaughlin, 1994, Employment, unemployment and social security, in A. Glyn and D. Miliband, *Paying for Inequality*, London: Institute for Public Policy Research.
49 A.B. Atkinson and G. Mogensen, 1993, *Welfare and Work Incentives*, Oxford: Clarendon.
50 D. Gallie, C. Marsh and C. Vogler (eds), 1994, *Social Change and the Experience of Unemployment*, Oxford: Oxford University Press.
51 A. Gouldner, 1960, The norm of reciprocity, *American Sociological Review*, 25(2), 161–77; A. Heath, 1976, *Rational Choice and Social Exchange*, Cambridge: Cambridge University Press.
52 R. Walker, 1994, *Poverty Dynamics*, Aldershot: Avebury.
53 P. Buhr and S. Leibfried, 1995, What a difference a day makes: the significance for social policy of the duration of social assistance receipt, in G. Room (ed.), 1995, *Beyond the Threshold*, Bristol: Policy Press.
54 L. Morris, 1994, *Dangerous Classes: The Underclass and Social Citizenship*, London: Routledge.
55 S. Mennell, 1974, *Sociological Theory*, London: Thomas Nelson, Ch. 5.
56 G. Varnava, 1995, Do be careful kids, it's a jungle outside, *Sunday Times*, 1 October, 6.
57 G. Himmelfarb, 1995, The value of Victorian virtues, *Sunday Times*, 16 April, 3.
58 S. Box, 1987, *Recession, Crime and Punishment*, London: Macmillan.
59 J. Young, 1986, Recent developments in criminology, in M. Haralambos, *Developments in Sociology*, Ormskirk: Causeway Books.
60 G. Sorel, 1961, *Reflections on Violence*, New York: Collier-Macmillan.
61 W. Thomas and F. Znaniecki, 1920, *The Polish Peasant in Europe and America*, Chicago: Chicago University Press.

13 The economy

1 R. Rose, 1984, *Understanding Big Government*, London: Sage.
2 M. Todaro, 1994, *Economic Development*, New York: Longmans, pp.160–3.
3 M. Andries, 1996, The politics of targeting: the Belgian case, *Journal of European Social Policy*, 6(3), 209–23.
4 Z. Bauman, 1997, *Postmodernity and its Discontents*, Oxford: Blackwell, p.36.
5 U. Beck, 1996, *Reflexive Modernisation*, Oxford: Polity Press; U. Beck, 1997, *Reinventing Politics*, Oxford: Polity Press.

6 M. Mullard, 1997, The politics of public expenditure control: a problem of politics or language games? *Political Quartery*, 68(3), 266–76.

14 The political framework

1 J. Drèze and A. Sen, 1989, *Hunger and Public Action*, Oxford: Clarendon Press.
2 R. Nozick, 1974, *Anarchy, State and Utopia*, Oxford: Blackwell, p.30.
3 R. Bernstein, 1991, *The New Constellation: the Ethical-Political Horizons of Modernity/Post Modernity*, Cambridge: Polity Press, p.336.
4 N. Bobbio, 1987, *The Future of Democracy*, Cambridge: Polity.
5 A. Heller, 1990, *Can Modernity Survive?*, Oxford: Polity Press, p.368.
6 S. Bowles and H. Gintis, 1986, *Democracy and Capitalism*, London: Routledge and Kegan Paul, p.186.
7 J. Shklar, 1989, The liberalism of fear, in N. Rosenblum, *Liberalism and the Moral Life*, London: Harvard University Press, p.15.
8 Heller, 1990, p.368.
9 Heller, 1987, p.163.
10 B. Barber, 1984, *Strong Democracy*, Berkeley: University of California Press.
11 P. Hansen, 1993, *Hannah Arendt: Politics, History and Citizenship*, Cambridge: Polity Press.
12 G. Sartori, 1987, *The Theory of Democracy Revisited*, Chatham, NJ: Chatham House, p.18.
13 A. Arblaster, 1987, *Democracy*, Buckingham: Open University Press.
14 Sartori, 1987.
15 Sartori, 1987, p.8.
16 P. Spicker, 1984, *Stigma and Social Welfare*, Beckenham: Croom Helm.
17 See e.g. J. Edwards, 1994, Group rights versus individual rights: the case of race-conscious policies, *Journal of Social Policy*, 23(1), 55–70; J. Crawford (ed.), 1988, *The Rights of Peoples*, Oxford: Clarendon Press.
18 A. Briggs, 1961, The welfare state in historical perspective, *European Journal of Sociology*, 2, 221–58.

15 Social welfare and social justice

1 Plato, *The Republic*.
2 J. Rawls, 1971, *A Theory of Justice*, Oxford: Oxford University Press.
3 Commission on Social Justice, 1994, *Social Justice*, London: Vintage.
4 J.A.K. Thomson, 1953, *The Ethics of Aristotle*, Harmondsworth: Penguin.
5 R. Nozick, 1974, *Anarchy, State and Utopia*, Oxford: Blackwell.
6 F. Hayek, 1976, *Law, Legislation and Liberty, Vol. 2: The Mirage of Social Justice*, London: Routledge and Kegan Paul.
7 H.B. Acton, 1971, *Morals of Markets*, London: Longman; B. de Jouvenel, 1951, *Ethics of Redistribution*, Cambridge: Cambridge University Press.
8 J. Rawls, 1971, *A Theory of Justice*, Oxford: Oxford University Press.

9 Rawls, 1971, p.199.
10 N. Daniels, 1975, *Reading Rawls*, Oxford: Blackwell.
11 R. Dworkin, 1985, *A Matter of Principle*, Cambridge, Mass.: Harvard University Press, p.192.
12 R.M. Titmuss, 1968, *Commitment to Welfare*, London: George Allen and Unwin.
13 S.I. Benn and R.S. Peters, 1959, *Social Principles and the Democratic State*, London: Allen and Unwin.
14 D. Rae, 1981, *Equalities*, Cambridge, Mass.: Harvard University Press.
15 J.H. Schaar, 1971, Equality of opportunity, and beyond, in A. de Crespigny and A. Wertheimer (eds), *Contemporary Political Theory*, London: Nelson.
16 Rae, 1981.
17 R. Carr-Hill, 1987, The inequalities in health debate, *Journal of Social Policy*, 16(4), 509–42; P. Townsend, N. Davidson and M. Whiteread, 1988, *Inequalities in Health*, Harmondsworth: Penguin; but see R. Illsley, J. Le Grand and C. Mullings, 1991, *Regional Inequalities in Mortality*, London: LSE Welfare State Programme.
18 A.B. Atkinson, A. Maynard and C. Trinder, 1983, *Parents and Children*, London: Heinemann; I. Kolvin, F. Miller, D. Scott, S. Gatzanis and M. Fleeting, 1990, *Continuities of Deprivation?*, Aldershot: Avebury.
19 R. Walker, 1995, The dynamics of poverty and social exclusion, in G. Room (ed.), *Beyond the Threshold*, Bristol: Policy Press.
20 Personal communication.
21 V. George, 1988, *Wealth, Poverty and Starvation*, Brighton: Wheatsheaf, p.208.
22 M. Baratz and W. Grigsby, 1971, Thoughts on poverty and its elimination, *Journal of Social Policy*, 1(2), 119–34.
23 F. Coffield and J. Sarsby, 1980, *A Cycle of Deprivation?*, London: Heinemann; I. Kolvin, F. Miller, D. Scott, S. Gatzanis and M. Fleeting, 1990, *Continuities of Deprivation?*, Aldershot: Avebury.
24 G. Simmel, 1908, The Poor, trans. C. Jacobson, *Social Problems*, 1965, 13 (Fall), 118–39.
25 M. O'Higgins and S. Jenkins, 1990, Poverty in the European Community, in R. Teekens and B. van Praag (eds), *Analysing Poverty in the European Community*, Eurostat News Special Edition, Luxembourg: EC.
26 Economic and Social Consultative Assembly, 1989, Ch. 7.
27 R. Lenoir, 1974, *Les Exclus*, Paris: Editions du Seuil.
28 P. Spicker, 1995, Inserting the excluded: the impact of the Revenu Minimum d'Insertion on poverty in France, *Social Work in Europe*, 22, 8–14.
29 Rae, 1981.
30 e.g. R. Dworkin, 1978, *Taking Rights Seriously*, London: Duckworth.
31 J. Edwards, 1987, *Positive Discrimination, Social Justice and Social Policy*, London: Tavistock.
32 J. Le Grand, 1982, *The Strategy of Equality*, London: Allen and Unwin.
33 G. Bramley and G. Smart, 1993, *Who Benefits from Local Services?*, LSE/STICERD.

34 R.M. Titmuss, 1995, The social division of welfare: some reflections on the search for equity, in *Essays on 'the Welfare State'*, 2nd edn 1963, London: George Allen and Unwin.
35 K. Boulding, 1973, The boundaries of social policy, in W.D. Birrell, P.A.R. Hillyard, A.S. Murie and D.J.D. Roche (eds), *Social Administration: Readings in Applied Social Science*, Harmondsworth: Penguin, p.192.
36 Cited J. Greve, 1975, Comparisons, perspectives, values, in E. Butterworth and R. Holman (eds), *Social Welfare in Modern Britain*, Glasgow: Collins, pp.184–5.
37 See P. Spicker, 1995, *Social Policy: Themes and Approaches*, Hemel Hempstead: Prentice Hall/Harvester Wheatsheaf, Ch. 5.
38 Tawney, 1931, p.56.
39 The *Guardian*, 1996, The end of the welfare state, 8 May, p.1.
40 R. Goodin and J. Le Grand (eds), 1987, *Not Only the Poor*, London: Allen and Unwin.

Index